THE **HAND** BOOK

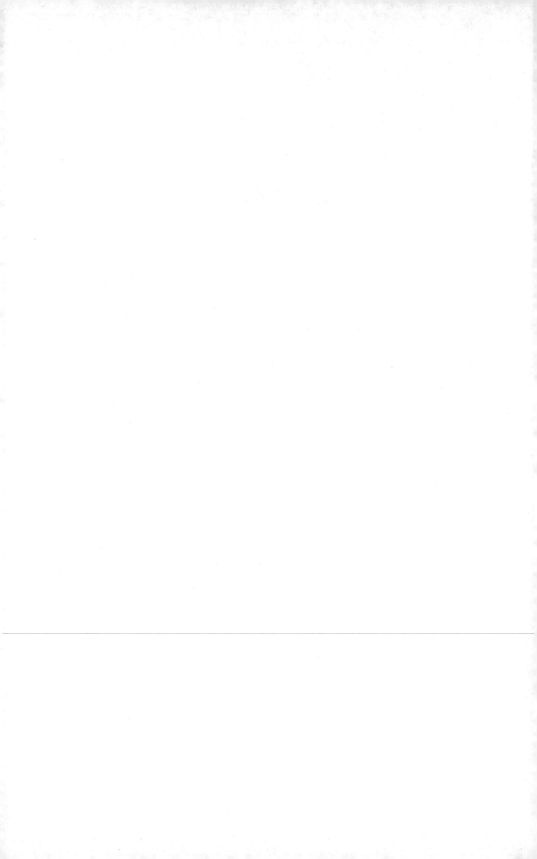

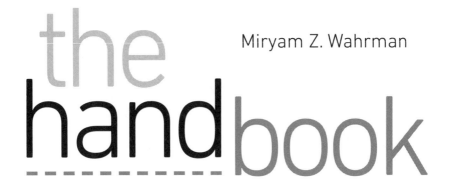

Miryam Z. Wahrman

the hand book

SURVIVING IN
A GERM-FILLED
WORLD

ForeEdge

ForeEdge
An imprint of University Press of New England
www.upne.com
© 2016 Miryam Z. Wahrman
All rights reserved
Manufactured in the United States of America
Designed by Eric M. Brooks
Typeset in Arnhem by Passumpsic Publishing

For permission to reproduce any of the material in this
book, contact Permissions, University Press of New England,
One Court Street, Suite 250, Lebanon NH 03766;
or visit www.upne.com

Library of Congress Cataloging-in-Publication Data
Names: Wahrman, Miryam Z., 1956–
Title: The hand book: surviving in a germ-filled world / Miryam Z. Wahrman.
Description: Lebanon, NH: ForeEdge, an imprint of University Press of New
    England, 2016. | Includes bibliographical references and index.
Identifiers: LCCN 2015034478 (print) | LCCN 2015044098 (ebook) |
    ISBN 9781611689174 (cloth) | ISBN 9781611685244 (pbk.) |
    ISBN 9781611689556 (ebook) | ISBN 9781611689556 (epub, pdf & mobi)
Subjects: LCSH: Hygiene. | Hand washing. | Hand—Care and
    hygiene. | Cross infection—Prevention.
Classification: LCC RA780 .W34 2016 (print) | LCC RA780 (ebook) |
    DDC 613—dc23
LC record available at http://lccn.loc.gov/2015034478

5 4 3 2 1

To my inspirations from the past,
ZEV AND EDITH ZAHAVY,
of blessed memory

To my inspirations who give me hope for the future,
ABBY, ELIYAHU, ILANA, ATARA, & NOAM COOPER
SUSIE AND MIKE RATNER

To my inspiration for life,
ISRAEL WAHRMAN

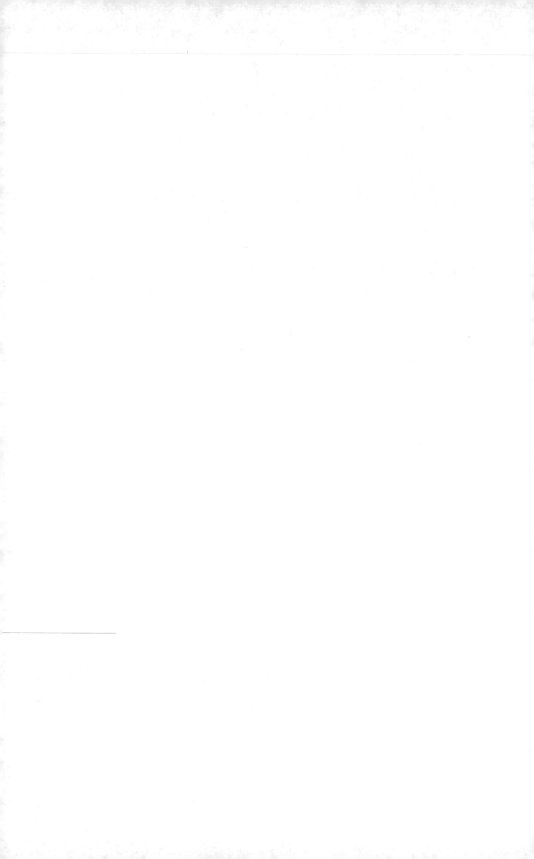

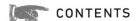 CONTENTS

HANDY LISTS

Hands Can Be Hazardous to Your Health

Germs know no borders. They cross continents and oceans, carried by infected individuals just a plane ride away. Outbreaks of disease happen all the time in various corners of the world. Many people fear that it is just a matter of time before an outbreak in one area becomes an epidemic, and then a pandemic, as travelers bring germs from place to place, from country to country. In my lifetime, worldwide epidemics of Asian flu, cholera, and mumps have occurred. Outbreaks of Ebola, measles, plague, SARS, malaria, polio, smallpox (yes, smallpox!), hepatitis B, meningitis, yellow fever, and other deadly diseases also have occurred among populations and in areas that seem far away, but are no longer isolated from us. "It's a Small World After All" is not just a jaunty Disney song; it's a warning that infectious diseases in one region can threaten the world population.

As scary as they seem, exotic diseases in remote places are not the ones that pose the biggest threats. Infectious diseases at home and in our healthcare settings are hazardous to our health on a day-to-day basis. How can we protect ourselves from dangerous infectious diseases that kill and maim millions in the United States and worldwide? One approach that reduces the risk of contracting many infectious diseases is the simple act of handwashing. Wherever you are, whether at home or abroad, washing your hands can lower your risk of infection. Hand hygiene can stem the tide of many diseases and slow their spread. Handwashing helps to keep travelers safe. Hand hygiene reduces the transmission of disease and the number of victims in homes, schools, workplaces, hospitals, clinics, and other healthcare settings.

I have been asked why I wanted to write a book about handwashing. After all, most of us do not contract deadly infectious diseases most of the time. We have evolved barriers and immune mechanisms that protect us. However, we need to be prepared for the inevitable—that we will be exposed to infectious agents that cause disease, and that germs from other people, perhaps our neighbors, or from other parts of the world, will find their way to our communities, and to us, and endanger our lives. Local, homegrown outbreaks of antibiotic-resistant bacteria pose a significant threat to health. Drug-resistant bacteria can originate in clinics and hospital wards, and spread through the vulnerable patient population and beyond. Some of the time, in particular in vulnerable hospital patients, the protective mechanisms—skin, mucous, tears, immune system—will fail to protect us, leaving us susceptible to disease. One effective approach to reducing risk is to remain vigilant and reduce the opportunities for germs to breach our defenses. The first line of defense is keeping our hands clean.

In a way, I have been preparing to write this book throughout my life. I was raised in a household by parents who were, to put it mildly, hygiene conscious. My father, in particular, was extra cautious about germs. When I was a child, my father showed my brothers and me how to open public doors by using a tissue (we called them Kleenexes) to turn the doorknob. When we went to a public bathroom, he instructed us "put down paper" before sitting down, and we were taught to flush "touchless style," to use a paper towel to turn on and off the water and to exit the facility without ever touching a public surface. When we traveled, my dad would "alcoholize" surfaces in the hotel room. The toilet, the phone, and other things we might touch were wiped down with ethyl alcohol that he always carried in a discreet bottle in his luggage. When alcohol wipes came out for personal use, he purchased boxes of them. We were the original "germies," or germaphobes, always on alert for situations that might expose us to public germs. To this day I carry a small bottle of alcohol in my travel case.

As a child, I loved animals and was curious about nature. I spent long summer afternoons swimming in the ocean and wandering down the beach, picking up shells and clams and crabs. I had opportunities to play with my older brothers' chemistry sets and microscopes, which opened a new world to me. And the Apollo moon missions further inspired me, and a whole generation of kids, to love science. Television coverage of space travel brought scientific exploration into our living room and made science seem exciting and mysterious.

I studied biology in college, and went on to earn my Ph.D. in biochemistry, studying cancer cells growing "in vitro," in laboratory dishes.[1] My research on cancer cells necessitated my becoming a "germie" in my professional life, and I was trained to maintain germfree surfaces and became an expert on aseptic—germfree—technique. This was crucial to my research, since I needed to maintain the cancer cells growing germfree for many years.[2] I learned the best approaches for keeping materials and the environment sterile. I also rediscovered my love for peering at cells in the microscope and through that experience got a unique perspective on the world. When you use a microscope, wherever you look there is life. You can find microorganisms that inhabit every surface and nook and cranny on our fertile planet. The microscopic view of life reinforced my interest in microbes and my desire to understand how cells of all kinds survive and grow.

As a postdoctoral scientist, I tinkered with life, and genetically engineered bacterial cells to produce a set of microbes that carried human colon cancer genes. Those bacteria were used to study how cancer cells differ from normal cells.[3] The project also gave me experience handling and growing bacteria in the lab and using them as tools for cancer research.

Then a unique opportunity presented itself. I was hired to set up the In Vitro Fertilization Laboratory at Mount Sinai Medical Center. Since it was only a few years after the birth of Louise Brown, the world's first test-tube baby, it was a challenge to design and equip a laboratory to culture human eggs and to fertilize, nourish, and grow human embryos. My experience with aseptic cell culture was invaluable as the human eggs, sperm, and embryos had to be kept germfree, and alive and well, in artificial culture vessels. In addition, I had conducted research on sperm,[4] and that experience also helped prepare me for the challenges posed by IVF in the early 1980s. I was gowned and gloved each time I attended an egg-retrieval procedure in the operating room and excitedly waited to receive my tiny charges, the harvested eggs. I transported the eggs to the embryo lab for processing, mixed them with sperm, and nurtured the fertilized eggs and embryos as they developed, until they were ready to return to the womb.

Each egg and embryo was precious and irreplaceable, so we had to ensure the highest quality of care in a germfree environment. I published a paper on human egg pathology, one of the first to analyze the characteristics of normal and defective human eggs, with the goal of improving the success of the procedure.[5] When the first New York State test-tube baby was conceived in our embryo lab, my microphotographs of the embryos were widely disseminated. At Mount Sinai, I also conducted research on mouse embryo fertilization, where I fashioned tiny microneedles and pipets to mechanically inject sperm into eggs.[6] That project contributed to the development of human intracytoplasmic sperm injection (ICSI), a technique that is now used commonly in IVF when the male partner makes too few sperm.

I moved on to become professor of biology at William Paterson University, where I helped develop one of the first biotechnology programs in the world.[7] We brainstormed and invented courses that involved teaching new areas that were just emerging, such as applying DNA technology, studying proteins, and growing cells in culture. I helped to set up the laboratories and lab exercises for these courses, and taught sections of most of the new courses. Teaching cell culture to undergraduates and graduate students was challenging, as keeping the cells' environment germfree is not a skill that comes naturally to most people. We taught (and still teach) students biotechnology and aseptic technique and how to use cell culture as a tool to study many biological processes and problems.

I continued to pursue research in the areas of developmental biology, biochemistry,[8] and research on anticancer substances,[9] and in projects that involved culturing cells from insects,[10] frogs,[11] and mammals, and keeping those cells germfree. I also spent time directing the graduate program, chairing the Department of Biology, directing the university's general education program, and developing new curricula in biology and general education. I developed a broad, multidisciplinary outlook that gave me the opportunity to consider the bigger picture, which led me to consider, investigate, and write about issues in bioethics.[12] In 1997 I became science correspondent for the *New Jersey Jewish Standard* and wrote, and continue to write extensively, on science, health, bioethics, and religion.

In my book *Brave New Judaism: When Science and Scripture Collide*,[13] I explore Jewish bioethics, specifically how the Jewish faith addresses the use of new technologies. At William Paterson I developed curricula—workshops and courses in bioethics, including a graduate course, "Bioethics and Society," which I teach every year. In this course we tackle beginning and end-of-life issues, bioethics principles in health care, and how new technologies can lead to new bioethics dilemmas. I initiated a new microbiology research program, where I studied the contamination of men's neckties with bacteria and went on to explore the interaction of bacteria with other surfaces found in clinical environments, such as fabrics, latex, and hard surfaces. I teach students who work in my lab how to maintain germfree conditions, test for bacterial contamination, and sterilize contaminated surfaces.

From a personal perspective, in addition to being raised a "germie," I also practiced good hand hygiene as a mother, raising healthy children, who were not by any stretch germfree, but are germ-aware. Now, as a grandmother, I get to experience cute grimy little hands again, and one of my goals is to pass on our family tradition of good hand hygiene.

In reaction to recent outbreaks of infectious disease, devices have been invented and installed in bathrooms to protect people from contamination. A visit to a public bathroom can be an adventure in modern electronics. There may be a button to open the door, an electric eye to flush the toilet, an automatic faucet, an electronic paper towel dispenser, and a jet-air dryer to dry hands without a need to touch the device. With these devices, it would appear that we already have solutions to the problem of hand hygiene. The electronic bathroom should protect us against biological hazards that could spread disease in public places. But the situation is far more complex, and hand hygiene still remains a major issue in public health and personal safety. Germs abound and health hazards are numerous and can be life threatening. Hospitals are experiencing crises as nosocomial, or hospital-acquired infections, sicken millions of patients each year and take the lives of tens of thousands.

When my mother entered the hospital with symptoms of a heart attack, the doctors recommended bypass surgery. She came through the surgery well and was beginning to recover. Then she suffered a serious setback— an infection in the sternal wound, the muscles and rib area that they cut open to reach her heart. This infection led to further surgery to cut away the infected tissue. Eventually, the infection spread to other body systems; and after a valiant struggle, over five-and-a-half months in the ICU, she passed away. It might seem far-fetched that a patient entering the hospital for one disease succumbs to another, completely unrelated one. But researchers have estimated that 5 to 10 percent of hospitalized patients contract hospital-acquired infections; this may involve up to two million patients, leading to ninety thousand deaths and a preventable cost of several billions of dollars.[14]

The same complication that killed my mother, an infection of the sternum, was reported in six British patients who had heart surgery, and the medical journal account unfolds like a CSI episode.[15] The first two cases appeared in March 2003, when doctors noted that after heart surgery two patients had complications. Upon investigation they determined that the same bacterial species, *Serratia marsescens*, was found in the wounds. Further testing of the bacteria showed that it was likely that they came from the same source. Two months later another case of a similar nature occurred in that hospital, which was also a match. The evidence for a single source of infection mounted, so the British Health Protection Agency Laboratory got involved. Using a more sensitive DNA test, they confirmed that in all three cases the bacteria came from the same source. Within months another three cases of sternal infections arose, bringing the total to six patients infected with the same deadly germs. Now a major health concern for the hospital, the source of the infection had to be found and stopped. But where could all six patients have acquired the same germs?

Medical detectives in the hospital tested the surgical suites, including the surfaces and air in the operating and anesthetic rooms that were used for all six operations, but those tests came up clean—no sign of that bacterial strain. Next they decided to screen the personnel involved in the surgeries. It turned out that two individuals, a nurse and an assisting surgeon, were present at all six surgeries, but initial screening of the two came up negative; there was no sign of the bacteria *S. marcessans* on either one. However, further questioning of the surgeon revealed that the doctor always wore two rings that were stuck on his fingers and never taken off. He had worn those rings, under his sterile glove, at all the surgeries. The skin under the rings was sampled and shown to harbor the same bacterial strain that was proven to have caused the infections in the six patients. The surgeon's rings were the culprits.[16]

How could such a mishap occur? It turns out that the physician was adhering to hospital policy, which permitted wedding bands to be worn in the operating room under sterile gloves. Studies have shown that people who wear rings can harbor higher levels of bacteria on their hands, trapped beneath their rings, and there are a number of reports of glove breakage during cardiac surgery; therefore, it should not be a surprise that contaminated rings can lead to infected patients. Although he had scrubbed and gloved for surgery, the bacteria found its way from his rings into patient incisions and infected them. The paper concludes, "We feel that this unusual outbreak adds further weight to the recommendation that finger rings should be removed prior to scrubbing." And the fate of that surgeon? He was not permitted to perform surgery again until he had his rings removed and passed three successive screening tests to show that he had eliminated those germs from his hands. When he was finally cleared, he was able to resume operating.[17]

Did my mother die because of a similar preventable lapse of hygiene? We will never know for sure, but perhaps we can learn a lesson about the critical importance of hygiene from her death, and the preventable deaths of other patients.

Hand hygiene can be a life-and-death issue in hospitals, but it also sickens people in other settings on a daily basis, when germs are transferred from person to person, from hands to surfaces and back again to hands. Many in the food industry have changed their practices when handling food and some of these changes have been legislated. The Pennsylvania Food Code states: "Food employees may not wear jewelry (including medical information jewelry) on their arms and hands while preparing food. This prohibition does not apply to a plain ring such as a wedding band."[18] The code also specifies how to wash hands, arms, and fingernails and requires workers to cover their hair. When adhered to, even flawed legislation can reduce the risk of food-borne illness. (Of course, we know this particular policy is flawed, considering that disease germs could be hiding under wedding rings.)

Some food establishments make their workers wear disposable gloves or pick up the food items indirectly—for instance, with tongs or a piece of wax paper. But the laws and policies are far from perfect; food workers may fail to comply or may go through the motions in an inadequate manner because they do not understand the mechanism of contamination. I have often observed a food worker serve food, take money, use the cash register, give change, scratch his or her face, adjust hair, and go on to serve the next customer, all with the same pair of gloves. The germaphobe in me cringes.

Years ago whenever our father gave us kids, and later on his grandkids, money for a special occasion, he would first go to the bank and request new bills so he would be able to give out the cleanest and crispest currency.

Without having looked into a microscope, my father knew that money harbors germs, and paper money is an excellent vector for all sorts of microbes. Some people touch their money after coughing and sneezing or after going to the bathroom, and bacteria and viruses can survive for days or weeks on paper money. One study showed that 94 percent of dollar bills collected in western Ohio were contaminated with bacteria. Seven percent of the bills had germs that could cause serious disease.[19] Do we need to wash our hands every time we touch money? That would be one approach, but not a practical one. Fortunately, our skin does protect us from exposure to many of the germs we encounter, so we do not have to wash all the time. But it does make sense to wash hands well before eating, after using the bathroom, and before touching the mouth, nose, or eyes.

There are many choices of cleansers for handwashing. It can seem overwhelming to buy hand soap or cleansers because there are so many (too many?) choices: bar soap, liquid soap, antibacterial soap with triclosan or other chemicals, body washes, and detergents. What cleansers work best? This question is not that simple to answer. Research done in my lab at William Paterson University has shown that antimicrobial soaps with triclosan do kill some bacteria, but do not completely sanitize. Other soaps and washes have an even more limited effect on bacteria. In our experiments the most effective antibacterials turned out to be 70 percent ethyl alcohol or 3 percent hydrogen peroxide. Products such as alcohol-based Purell really do work to kill bacteria. So my father's approach of using alcohol to disinfect was, after all, a wise one.

But you do not have to squirt your hands with alcohol all day to stay healthy. Regular soaps work well because, even though those products do not kill many germs, they wash dirt and germs off of the surface of your hands, and that appears to be effective enough to keep most people healthy. In fact, there is something to be said for preserving some of the native bacteria on our skin, our so-called "microbiome." We harbor populations of harmless bacteria all over our bodies. These good bacteria populate the skin and inhabit niches, typically outcompeting disease-causing bacteria, so we would not want to remove all the bacteria in our environment. There have been concerns that the overuse of antimicrobial chemicals can reduce the population of harmless bacteria, providing opportunities for pathogenic (disease-causing) bacteria to thrive.

Common objects also can be a source for the spread of disease. Cell phones, handbags, doorknobs, and other people's hands can spread infections and lead to contamination and disease. But it is impractical to suggest that we refrain from touching anything or that we cover our hand with a tissue before touching every surface. We need to be aware of how environmental surfaces can transmit germs and act accordingly.

One area for reducing risk is by controlling contamination on healthcare workers' clothing. The necktie, in particular, can be a culprit in spreading germs because it is a garment worn over and over, day after day, and rarely cleaned. Research in my laboratory has shown that necktie fabrics can be contaminated with various types of bacteria, and the bacteria can survive for long periods of time on the material. Silk appears to harbor more germs and be more resistant to cleansing than polyester. Bacteria also adhere well to cotton and wool. Certain types of microfiber do not harbor many bacteria as they are hydrophobic and repel water, or anything with polar or charged surfaces, like microbes. This research can help generate guidelines for healthcare workers to reduce contamination. When there was an outbreak of MRSA (methicillin-resistant *Staphylococcus aureus*) in 2006, doctors in the United Kingdom were advised by the British Medical Association to stop wearing neckties. This sort of policy has not been common in the United States, but observations and data from my laboratory could encourage doctors and other healthcare professionals to follow suit.

Our attitudes on hand hygiene can affect how well we manage the risks associated with disease-causing microorganisms. It is important to consider culture as well as the history of hand hygiene to understand what practices are the most critical to keep us healthy. There are thousands of years of human history in which people survived without electric sinks, automatic toilets, and antibacterial soaps. This historical perspective can illuminate how people stayed healthy before high-tech hygiene was invented and can give us insight into what may be important in our current practices. For instance, in Leviticus 15:11 the Bible states that if a man who has a "running issue out of his flesh" (usually interpreted as a contagious sexually transmitted disease, possibly gonorrhea) touches someone "without having rinsed his hands in water," the person who has been touched will become unclean. The required purification includes washing clothes, bathing in water, rinsing hands in water, washing wooden vessels, and destroying clay vessels touched by the patient. It appears that thousands of years ago religious dictates required handwashing and other hygienic practices to address disease.

Cultural differences in hand hygiene are also helpful in understanding how to reduce risk. Japanese attitudes on hygiene differ dramatically from those of Western cultures. Handshaking, a common Western behavior, is not practiced in the Japanese culture. As we learn about hand hygiene in other parts of the world, we may want to adopt some foreign practices that appear to reduce the risk of transmitting disease. Culture drives behavior, and in Western culture failing to shake hands in social situations could be construed as an insult. But in consideration of the health of his guests, Jon Stewart of *The Daily Show* made a point of replacing handshakes with elbow bumps when he was suffering from a bad cold.

In the course of writing this book, I have been reflecting on hands and their roles in our lives and in human history. Human hands make us uniquely human. They provide us with special abilities far beyond those of other animals. We use our hands to make tools, and although there are other primates that use tools, we humans do it to a greater degree. We also use hands to fashion art, and to perform musically, clapping, drumming, and strumming. The word root *art* refers to that which is made by human hands and ingenuity (artisan, artistic, artifact, and artificial refer to the producers, process, and products of human hands). Our talented hands are also used in written expression—another uniquely human accomplishment. Our hands write, paint, sculpt, make music, and greet each other, in a distinctly human fashion. People ask me why I wrote a book about handwashing and whether there is enough to say to fill a whole book. Well, yes there is, and then some. And all of it is relevant and important to anyone who has hands or knows someone who does.

I want to add a note about the term *handwashing*. There is no such word in the English lexicon, as the official term is *hand washing*. But just as *hand* and *shake* go together in a friendly *handshake*, *hands* and *washing* are partners in *handwashing*, an act that is beneficial and health promoting. In fact, *handwashing* already is an accepted term, as the Centers for Disease Control and Prevention uses *handwashing*, as do many professional journals. There is a Global Handwashing Day (October 15) and a National Handwashing Awareness Week (mid-December). The goal of this book is to change the culture and attitudes making handwashing a routine and expected behavior. In the process of conveying this message, perhaps we can change the lexicon as well to accept *handwashing* as part of our official language, as well as our healthier lives.

In chapter 1, "Handwashing Habits, Hygiene, and Health," we begin our story of handwashing by exploring microbiomes, that is, the populations of microbes that live among us, and the relationships between humans and microorganisms, including benign ones that make up our normal flora and keep us healthy, and malevolent ones that can cause disease. I reveal who is washing or not washing hands, and how best to wash and dry hands. In chapter 2, "Microbe Hunting: Historic and Biological Roots of Hygiene," I look at how ancient cultures and communities dealt with disease and hygiene, how scientists' discoveries led to the development of the germ theory, and how the scientific heroes who laid the foundation for modern hygiene changed the playing field. Chapter 2 also explains the different types of germs and microbes and how unhygienic habits can pose a threat to the human population. Chapter 3, "First Do No Harm," investigates hand hygiene in clinical settings, and how lapses in hygiene by doctors, nurses, and other healthcare professionals can lead to medical complications and death. In chapter 4, "Touch at Your Own Risk," I examine how microbes found on environmental surfaces can transmit disease. Germs from an infected person can contaminate everyday objects and be passed to another person, leading to infection. Chapter 5, "Solutions: Protecting Ourselves and Society," offers solutions and strategies to reduce the risk of infectious disease and decrease transmission from person to person. Finally, chapter 6, "The Future of Hand Hygiene: It's Not a Game," looks at the types of initiatives that offer hope to help humanity deal with ever more complex microbial issues, such as drug resistance and residing in a smaller interconnected world. This last chapter also provides practical advice for hand hygiene and reducing infection.

I have been thinking about and practicing the principles of hand hygiene for as long as I can remember, in my personal and professional lives. I have thought long and hard about the practical issues of hand hygiene as an approach to reducing the risk of disease. I demonstrate in this book that there are simple acts of hygiene that can protect us and keep us healthier. Not everyone subscribes to these principles or complies with these acts, and that can lead to the spread of disease and to death. The science is complex but the message is simple. The goal of *The Hand Book* is to serve as a road map to safer hands, better hygiene, better health, and a longer life.

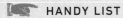 **HANDY LIST**

Germ-Laden Surfaces in Public Places

1. Sinks in public restrooms
2. Shopping cart handles
3. Playground swings and jungle gyms
4. Telephones and keyboards in the office
5. High chairs in restaurants
6. Cruise ship handrails
7. Bus and subway handrails
8. Escalator handrails in malls
9. ATM touch pads
10. Public pens and the credit-card machine stylus
11. Doorknobs
12. An open common bowl of mints, chips, nuts, pretzels
13. Money
14. Restaurant menus
15. Lemon wedges in restaurants
16. Airplane bathrooms
17. Doctors' offices

ACKNOWLEDGMENTS

I would not have been able to write this book if I had not been born to two amazing parents, who raised me to be inquisitive, confident, skeptical, and wary of germs. I am grateful to my parents, of blessed memory, for a loving home, and for their constant encouragement and support. My interest in science was ignited by my loving, resourceful, and patient mother; my role model, Edith Zahavy, with whom I conversed every day; and my brilliant, loving, generous, creative, unconventional father, Rabbi Dr. Zev Zahavy, who reinvented himself in middle age to become an English professor and cosmologist. My exceptional brothers, Rabbi Dr. Tzvee Zahavy and Professor Reuvain Zahavy, let me tag along with them throughout my childhood, including me in their adventures, inviting me into the tree house, and passing on their microscopes, chemistry sets, trains, and Lincoln Logs. My brothers grew up to be my dear friends, who are still role models, and people I consult and confer with over important issues. I thank Tzvee for encouraging me to write for America Online, for feedback on this book, and most important, for bringing Bernice Zahavy into our family—as she is a best friend and someone I can always count on.

I met my husband, Dr. Israel Wahrman, Esq., when I was seventeen, and two years later I was his teenage bride. We have been growing up together ever since. Traveling life's bumpy road with him has been a wonderful adventure, and his love and support have enabled me to achieve many dreams. He contributed tremendously to this project with sage advice and insightful feedback on the manuscript. He soars like an eagle in his own achievements, as a husband and father, in his career in psychology, as a midlife law student and now an administrative law judge. To him I owe my deepest love and gratitude, as well as pride in all he has accomplished.

On this bumpy road of life we have been blessed with tremendous joy and with loving family and friends. We were blessed with two delightful little girls, who washed their hands as needed and grew up into two beautiful, intelligent, and delightful women. I thank my dear daughters, Abigail Rebecca Cooper, M.D., and Susanna Wahrman Ratner, Esq., for their unwavering support and for critical reading of the manuscript. A doctor and a lawyer, what more could a mother want? Well, life just keeps on giving, and our daughters gave us two brilliant, kind, and caring sons-in-law, anesthesiologist Eliyahu Cooper, M.D., and mathematician Michael Ratner. And blessings continue to flow from above, in the form of three happy, energetic, and amazingly beautiful geniuses, Ilana Sophia, Atara Emma, and Noam Zev Cooper. And yes, I am allowed to be effusive and over the top, since they are my grandkids.

I have also been inspired by Rabbi Solomon and Sarah Wahrman, of blessed memory, both of whom published memoirs of their European childhoods and their Holocaust nightmares and survival. My father-in-law was a scholar and author who contributed greatly to the field of *halakha*, Jewish law. They were people of strength and substance, courage and conviction, who raised three fine sons. Jack and Fagie Wahrman and Chaim Dov and Breindy Wahrman have been caring and supportive sisters- and brothers-in-law through good as well as challenging times. I also thank two special friends, who are more like family, who are always there for me with encouragement and support, Dorothea Krieger and Peggy Cottrell.

I thank Hunter College of the City University of New York for a first-rate and free undergraduate education only one block from my home. At Cornell University Graduate School of Medical Sciences and Sloan-Kettering Institute I benefited greatly from the mentorship of Dr. Aaron Bendich, a renowned biochemist, and Dr. Leonard Augenlicht, who was a young and enthusiastic role model for me. He is now a highly accomplished biomedical scientist, who has contributed tremendously to our understanding of the molecular biology of cancer. I have received tremendous support from current and past colleagues at William Paterson University, in particular, those who worked with me on research projects: Professors Corey Basch, Eileen Gardner, Jaishri Menon, Gurdial Sharma, Joseph Spagna, and Jean Werth. Patricia Bush, Mukesh Sahni, Susan Sgro, and Michael Wyrwa have also provided helpful guidance. I thank Professor Robert Chesney for advice in microbiology when I launched a new research program, and for his critical review of this manuscript. My students who worked diligently on various microbiology projects include: Melanie Colon, Samantha Deceglie, Shamil Javed, Karina Kuruvilla, Brianna McSweeney, Brian Nelson, Shalaka Paranjpe, Jigna Patel, Henry Raab, Peter Rogers, Khushnuma Sabavala, Jay Shah, and Raahi Upadhyay. I received helpful input on religious ritual for this book from Joseph Spagna, Denise Liberty, and Nathan Lewis.

The administrators at William Paterson University continue to be motivating and supportive of research and scholarship by providing resources and release time. I thank President Kathleen Waldron, Provost Warren Sandmann, Dean Kenneth Wolf, Biology Chairperson David Slaymaker, and former Chair Lance Risley for their support and commitment to faculty and student research.

I thank my superb editor, Phyllis Deutsch, who is patient and encouraging; copyeditor Elizabeth Forsaith for polishing and clarifying the text; and the rest of the staff at University Press of New England/ForeEdge, who produce an impressive array of amazing books. I am grateful to my agent, Joseph Spieler, for his valuable guidance and advice. I owe a debt of gratitude to Rebecca Boroson, retired editor of the *New Jersey Jewish Standard*, who was a tremendous force in molding me as a science correspondent, and I thank Joanne Palmer, current editor, for producing a fine newspaper that I am proud to be a part of.

I am at the point in life where I can synthesize many of my personal and professional life experiences into a story that teaches, from many perspectives, how to live a safer life by washing hands. I hope that my passion for hand hygiene leads to a better appreciation of science and health and a world that is safer and healthier. I express regrets for any errors, omissions, or misstatements. Now I respectfully advise you to go wash your hands.

MZW, August 2015

Handwashing Habits, Hygiene, and Health

Despite all that we have learned from our parents and teachers, hygienic practices, including handwashing, can vary from person to person. Some people are scrupulous hand washers and others not so much. We like to believe that everyone washes their hands after using the bathroom and before eating, but research tells us otherwise. We can control our own behaviors and actions with regard to hygiene, but we cannot pretend that we know what other people do. We cannot impose our views on others (except perhaps our own small children) regarding even the simple act of handwashing. In fact, most of us—even dedicated germies—can still learn a thing or two about hygiene and can do better with regard to cleanliness. Even more so, people who have given the issue little thought may be able to learn a lot more about how to stay healthy in a germ-filled world. Because we are all interconnected, we are affected by how other people handle health care and hygiene.

Senator Thom Tillis, Republican from North Carolina, got his fifteen minutes of fame in early 2015 when he declared that restaurants should not be required to have their employees wash their hands after using the bathroom, as long as the restaurant posts a sign that they have no handwashing requirement. As a strong opponent of government regulations, Tillis defended this recommendation as an example of the way the free market should work. Businesses should be able to decide whether or not to require their employees to perform basic hygienic practices before handling customers' food, and customers (the free market at work) could then decide whether or not to patronize the restaurant. The Food and Drug Administration's (FDA's) view on the issue of hand hygiene for food handlers is clear: "Proper handwashing reduces the spread of fecal-oral pathogens from the hands of a food employee to foods."[1] Although he was subjected to the ridicule of late-night comics (Jon Stewart called him "Senator Dung-hands von Fecalfingers"), cable news pundits, and the print media, the senator did not later retract this controversial view, rather, he defended it in the name of freedom.

"It is absurd that the administration of a modern State should be left to men ignorant of science and of its human consequences," wrote Frederick Soddy, the 1921 Nobel laureate in chemistry.[2] This quote, which is as relevant today as it was almost a century ago, reflects the concern that politics can lead to policies that are inconsistent with science and potentially hazardous to individual and community health. Soddy lamented that the education system does not adequately prepare citizens to appreciate scientific research and what it can do for society. Nowadays we are still grappling with the lack of understanding and rejection of science. The scientific basis for hand hygiene provides us with valuable tools to reduce the incidence of disease and live healthier lives and should serve to guide policy and regulations.

The recent case of "the Senator versus handwashing regulations" demonstrates a misplaced faith in free-market capitalism, in which a politician expects free-market forces to close down dirty restaurants, or perhaps leave them open. Laissez-faire is simply not going to work in this case. Scientific research shows that many people do not even wash their own hands after using the bathroom, so the issue of what their waiter did or did not do may be totally off their radar. Consumers who are unaware that dirty hands can spread disease will not be concerned whether the food server has washed. People who do care may be too timid or embarrassed to ask a server to don disposable gloves or to use serving tongs instead of their hands. Perhaps some of them will walk out of the restaurant if there is a better option, but there may be no better restaurants to choose from in the neighborhood, as it is possible that all the area restaurants will adopt the laissez-faire attitude toward handwashing. If restaurants are not required to impose washing policies on their workers, many of the workers may not wash their hands.

The case of Typhoid Mary drives home the importance of the connection between hygiene and health in food establishments. From 1900 to 1907, Mary Mallon worked as a cook in New York City, but when she became infected with the *Salmonella enterica* bacteria (*S. typhi*), she transmitted typhoid fever to dozens of New Yorkers. An article published in *Cell Host & Microbe* clarifies how she could have been an asymptomatic carrier of the disease for so long.[3] This case was not an easy one to crack. It took years for authorities to make the connection between a series of outbreaks of the disease and the common factor, namely, the cook. When they found and arrested her, Mary Mallon admitted that she "rarely washed her hands."[4] This disease carrier did not, herself, get sick, but she was a vector for the disease. Many people, even food workers, are still unaware of the importance of handwashing, or simply refuse to do so, and are potential vectors for disease.

Hand Microbiomes
Communities of Microbes on Our Hands

The food-handler issue is one of concern, as we know from many studies that all humans carry a host of microorganisms on their hands. Many of the microbes are harmless flora that populate the skin and do not cause disease. But some are pathogens that transmit disease. Every nursing student is required to take a course in microbiology, where they may complete laboratory experiments that raise awareness of microbes and contamination, such as "Bacteria of the Skin," "Effectiveness of Hand Scrubbing," and "Chemical Methods of Control: Disinfectants and Antiseptics."[5] Students collect samples from their hands, arms, face, or leg, and culture them on nutrient agar petri dishes. They then identify the bacterial species using a battery of tests.

Bacteria typically found on skin include the resident, usually benign flora, such as *Staphylococcus epidermidis*, and the transient flora, which are picked up from other sources and can be pathogenic, such as potentially disease-causing *Staphylococcus aureus*. Although those two species of *Staphylococcus* share the same genus, they are very different in their potential to do harm. *S. aureus* is of concern as it can cause skin infections such as impetigo, boils, and abscesses. Some strains of *S. aureus* produce toxins that can cause food poisoning or toxic shock syndrome (TSS). Increased risk of TSS has been linked to the use of certain types of ultra-absorbent tampons, but some victims contract it through other routes of entry. For instance, Jim Henson, who created the Muppets, died of toxic shock syndrome, in his case caused by yet another bacterial species, *Streptococcus pyogenes*, the same organism responsible for strep throat. That very contagious microbe, which is also known as group A streptococcus, can on rare occasions cause pneumonia, or complications involving the lungs, kidneys, or liver.

Flesh-eating disease is a particularly dreaded condition that can be caused by microbes around us. Known medically as necrotizing fasciitis, it can be caused by many types of bacteria, including *S. aureus* and *Streptococcus*.[6] An article published in *Reader's Digest*, "To Survive Flesh-Eating Bacteria,"[7] documents how author Hampton Sides almost lost his arm, and potentially even his life, to the infection. These media reports of dramatic infectious diseases make people stand up and take notice of the perils of infectious microbes. Although they are rare, people do contract infections, where the bacteria produce deadly toxins that consume or destroy vital tissue. Some victims are treated and cured by deep debridement (removal) of the infected tissue, or by more drastic solutions such as the amputation of limbs. For some the infection has spread too far and has destroyed critical organs, and the patient cannot be saved. While these are uncommon, skin infections should not be taken lightly, as complications can ensue, and even simple cuts and injuries can lead to serious complications.

Many species of bacteria dwell on our skin; one study found that more than a thousand different species make up the human skin microbiome, the community of bacteria that live on our skin, all over the body. Scientist Elizabeth Grice and her collaborators catalogued the diverse community of bacteria on twenty different skin sites in healthy humans. Grice works at the National Human Genome Research Institute, where reading the DNA of different organisms helps answer many biological questions that were previously unapproachable. The report describes the skin as "an ecosystem" with communities of microbes living under different conditions in "physiologically and topographically distinct niches" on different parts of the body. "For example, hairy, moist underarms lie a short distance from smooth dry forearms, but these two niches are likely as ecologically dissimilar as rainforests are to deserts." By learning about the normal population of microbes in the "rainforests" and "deserts" of our skin, they hope to better understand "the delicate balance between skin health and disease."[8]

On the global scale, a study funded by the Bill and Melinda Gates Foundation surveyed microbes associated with sick children—kids in six developing countries who had diarrheal diseases. The study showed that children in Bangladesh, India, Kenya, Mali, Mozambique, and Pakistan contract many germs that cause illness in these populations; however, four of the microbes stood out as being the main causes of life-threatening infections: a protozoa (protist) called Cryptosporidium, the *Shigella* bacteria, an *E. coli* species that makes a particular toxin, and the rotavirus.[9] By gaining access to this type of information, it makes it possible to better intervene. For instance, by vaccinating against the rotavirus, many children can avoid the infection completely.

The Microbiome Era

The ability to survey microbiomes, that is, the complete populations of microbes in a region, has been a game changer. Characterizing microbiomes on the skin, in the gut, or in the mouth helps define the good and bad microbes that keep us healthy or make us sick. Microbiomes in our external environments—in our homes, offices, hospitals, or outside—can also determine whether we are exposed to helpful or harmful organisms.

The new technologies that enable microbiome surveys rely on reading the genetic sequence of variations on the rDNA gene, a form of which is found in every living thing. Every organism from the lowliest bacteria to the exalted *Homo sapiens* has rDNA, or ribosomal DNA, as it is necessary to build ribosomes, the protein factories of all cells. Variants in these and other essential genes can be used to categorize different versions, or phylotypes, in a population. (In the bacterial world *phylotypes* can refer to variants of microbes, many of which are so new to us that they have not yet been grown in the lab or named.) This approach works very well in the characterization of thousands of different phylotypes of bacteria found in a microbiome.

Children in Bangladesh and Pakistan contract and die from infectious diseases, as previously described, but in truth, you do not have to travel to exotic destinations to be exposed to deadly germs. If we just look in our own backyards, playgrounds, and subways, we will find plenty of bacteria and other contaminants.

California and Arizona researchers tested environmental surfaces in four U.S. cities: Chicago, Tucson, San Francisco, and Tampa. They sampled over one thousand surfaces found in shopping centers, offices, day-care centers, airports, movie theaters, restaurants, and on personal items, to determine the presence of fecal and total coliform bacteria, and components of blood, urine, and other bodily fluids. The highest levels of contamination were found in daycare centers (in 46 percent of samples taken from those sites) and on playground equipment (in 36 percent of samples). Runners-up were in shopping environments, where 21 percent of samples had contaminants; in miscellaneous activities, where 21 percent were contaminated; and on office surfaces, where 11 percent had contaminants. In order to determine the risk of transfer, that is, contaminants spreading from surfaces to people and back to surfaces, the researchers used a fluorescent tracer to invisibly mark surfaces; the study showed that the tracer chemical was transferred from the surfaces to 86 percent of exposed hands. In addition, 82 percent of participants found evidence of the tracer in their homes or on their personal belongings hours later. The results help us understand the relative levels of contamination of public surfaces, and that in particular (but not surprisingly) children's playground equipment is a "priority surface" for the potential spread of infectious diseases.[10]

THE OFFICE MICROBIOME

As anyone who works in an office knows, what goes around comes around. This is true for office politics, and likewise for office illnesses. "The constant influx of microbes brought in with office workers makes for a dynamic microbial environment," asserts a research article written by biologists from San Diego State University and the University of Arizona. Many workers spend eight or more hours per day in an office building, where they may share facilities such as computers, chairs, conference rooms, restrooms, break rooms, and other common areas. The shared spaces can harbor germs that people leave behind, which can be transmitted to others in the office. Office germs from ninety offices in New York, San Francisco, and Tucson were surveyed in the study, which used genetic sequencing and cell culturing to find the germs. Four hundred and fifty samples were taken from desktops, chairs, phones, keyboards, and computer mice. The researchers found evidence of bacteria from more than five hundred different genera, the most abundant being microbes associated with "human skin, nasal, oral, or intestinal cavities." Bacteria typically found in soils also were common, perhaps because of the presence of office plants or materials tracked in on shoes. The microbiomes of New York and San Francisco offices were indistinguishable, but the populations of microbes found in Tucson offices differed from the other two cities. Chairs and phones were more contaminated than the other three surfaces. A notable finding was that "surfaces in offices inhabited by men were consistently more contaminated than those of offices inhabited by women." The authors speculate that the gender-related differences may be due to different hygienic practices. "Men are known to wash their hands and brush their teeth less frequently than women, and are commonly perceived to have a more slovenly nature." But they also suggest that part of the difference is because of men's larger body size and "correspondingly greater skin surface area, as well as nasal and oral cavities," as more surface area provides more space for bacteria to colonize.[11]

BELLY BUTTON MICROBIOMES

You can survey and study bacteria on common surfaces or in places you might not typically think about, such as belly buttons. Dr. Noah Fierer, who considers himself a "natural historian of cooties," has embarked on a quest to define microbiomes in a variety of settings. In addition to his team of scientists and graduate students, this microbiologist from the University of Colorado at Boulder has enlisted an army of citizen microbiologists to help him achieve his goals.[12] In a project that seems like something cooked up by the science nerds/geniuses on TV's *Big Bang Theory*, citizen scientists were recruited by Fierer and his gang to participate in the nationwide "Belly Button Biodiversity" project. "The belly button is one of the habitats closest to us, and yet it remains relatively unexplored," states the published report. They sampled the belly button bacteria from over five hundred volunteers, some of whom were recruited at Darwin Day at the Museum of Natural Sciences in Raleigh, North Carolina. This large group of volunteers gave their informed consent to have their belly buttons swabbed with sterile cotton tips in the name of science.[13]

It turns out that there were, on average, 67 different bacterial phylotypes per belly button, totaling at least 2,368 different species of bacteria. This is similar to other studies that showed astronomical numbers and great diversity of bacterial species in skin microbiomes. "Our diversity of bacterial phylotypes was more than twice as great as the species diversity of, for example, North American birds . . . or ants."[14] Who knew that belly buttons could be so complicated?

HOME MICROBIOMES

Belly button bacteria may be interesting as an academic pursuit, but the bacteria in belly buttons are typically symbionts—they live in harmony with us and do not harm us. The belly button study is not as medically relevant as learning about bacteria in microbiomes that could make us sick. Fierer and collaborators went on to study the home environment, once again with the assistance of citizen scientists, in a project dubbed "The Wild Life of Our Home." The study of bacteria in the home environment is of interest because it has been only a few decades since we learned how to make homes that are well removed from nature, with HVAC systems and windows we rarely open. "Humans are unique in producing elaborate homes, structures that through time have become more discrete and isolated from the outdoor environment," write Dunn and his coworkers.[15]

Surveying nine locations in each of forty different homes in Raleigh-Durham, North Carolina, the researchers reported that each location had distinctly different bacterial communities, and there was variability from home to home.[16] This type of study of bacteria might be analogous to comparing people you find in one city to those you find in another. There might be similarities in some demographic categories, but there will be variability in the population of humans you find in the two cities.

Why would individual homes be so different from each other? Part of the answer lies in the environment around each house. It is obvious that microbes can get into a house even if you keep all the windows closed, as you still walk in the door and carry in the newspaper from the front lawn, the groceries, your kids, everything that has collected on your shoes and clothing and other belongings, as well as all the microbes you picked up that are now frolicking in your gut, in your blood, and on your skin and body openings. Some people reside in fairly closed environments that might appear to reduce the infiltration of microbes. But in fact, no human being is sterile, and we are all surrounded by a cloud of microbes, kind of like the cloud that hovers over the *Peanuts* character "Pigpen." Our personal cloud of microbes moves with us and leaves remnants wherever we go, leaving a trail of human-associated skin, gut, and mouth bacteria.

In our highly engineered artificial environment, we still find ourselves surrounded by a host of very small creatures: bacteria, fungi, protozoa, and slightly bigger creatures: mites, flies, mosquitoes, beetles, cockroaches, and other insects. In our environments there also may be rodents and other pests that share human domiciles. Some people have houseplants that alter the environment with their own microbial flora; they contribute to the microbial community with their soil and leaf bacteria. And it turns out that pets have an enormous influence on the microbial flora in our homes. In the "Wild Life of Our Home" study, the researchers discovered that there is a significant difference in microbiomes in homes with dogs compared to home without dogs; in those homes there is an additional set of microbes that are typically associated with dogs. (No significant differences were seen in homes with cats, but the authors explain that it could be because the sample size was low—only three homes sampled had cats but no dogs.)

The authors note that other research has shown that "individuals in homes with dogs might be less at risk for allergenic diseases."[17] Stimulating the immune system at an early age by being exposed to dog microbiomes could have a positive effect on health. This type of observation supports the notion that bacteria have an important role in our lives, and creating too sterile an environment may be to our detriment. Clearly not all microbes are created equal; some may be beneficial, indeed.

The microbiology of the indoors was the subject of a review article by Scott Kelley and Jack Gilbert, who describe the "built environment," or BE, as the "modern ecological habitat of *Homo sapiens sapiens*" (aka the subspecies of *Homo sapiens* that is limited to modern humans).[18] They explain that BEs have artificial niches, or microenvironments, that differ from natural environments, and these BEs can support distinctive combinations of microbial populations, including colonies of bacteria and fungi. "We share our living spaces with an immense diversity of microbial life, some potentially bad, others good, and most just along for the ride," explain Kelley and Gilbert.[19] Some of these habitats have microbes that colonize them mainly because human cells and tissues are shed in different places indoors, such as restrooms, classrooms, and offices. Some have to do with the modern devices we use, such as catheters, showerheads, and therapy pools. Specialized microenvironments include the aquarium filters in fish tanks and medical devices in neonatal intensive care units. In each microenvironment there is a different signature set of microbes. The authors point out that since "the BE can . . . be a source of microbes that colonize people, it is essential that we investigate 'who lives where' in the BE."[20] Information that can affect our health could include the fact that damp surfaces encourage the growth of fungi, that microbes from the human gut and vagina contribute to the restroom microbiome, and that animal inhabitants contribute significantly to BEs wherever animals are found.

A flowchart provided in that article shows the transmission routes of microbes in a hypothetical Built Environment. With human skin at its center, arrows indicate movement of microbes from skin to home surfaces. Other arrows show the transfer of microbes from soil to shoes to home to skin, from air to ventilation to dust to skin, from pets to skin, and from gut and vagina to restroom to skin. The major concern is how we pick up microbes from around us and how the "unseen majority" will affect human health. "Without a doubt," conclude the authors, "this new field of research will lead to discoveries that will change the way that we build, clean and live in our new ecosystem."[21]

THE NEW YORK SUBWAY MICROBIOME

If you want to find a "panoply of microorganisms,"[22] what better place to look than a transit system that serves 1.7 billion riders per year? A huge collaborative research project was undertaken by forty-six investigators from fourteen New York City–based institutions, as well as six other research centers, to survey the microbial species in the "largest mass-transit system in the world (by station count)," the New York City Subway system.[23] The study was conducted in order to establish a "baseline metagenomic map" of the subway flora. In other words, this research yields information on what is normally present in New York subways, a unique Built Environment (BE). Having a baseline of what is normally there could be helpful in the event of an outbreak of infectious disease, epidemic, or a bioterrorism incident.[24] The scope of the research article is impressive and worth delving into, as it gives a glimpse of the complexity of life, even in the bowels of the New York subways.

In a forensic-like sweep of the city, 1,457 DNA samples were collected from all of the active subway stations in the city, and from one closed subway station, looking for evidence of life below ground. (The South Ferry Station in lower Manhattan, which had been flooded during Superstorm Sandy in 2012 and was shut down because of extensive damage, was part of the project.) Subway station kiosks, benches, turnstiles, garbage cans, and railings were sampled. DNA analysis identified 1,688 different life forms. In chapter 2 we will discuss how the different living organisms are organized into domains and kingdoms; this survey found representatives from all three domains of life: eukaryotes, bacteria, and archaea.[25]

A whopping 48 percent of the DNA samples collected did not match sequences of any known organisms, suggesting that there is a "large, unknown catalog of life directly beneath our fingertips that remains to be discovered and characterized."[26] This is good news for biologists, who will not be running out of research subjects anytime soon.

The data showed that the busier the station was in terms of riders, the higher the diversity in terms of microbes. The major bacterial species found were those typically found on human skin, followed by bacteria of the gut and the urogenital tract. Of all the bacteria that were discovered, 57 percent were not disease causing and 31 percent were what is known as opportunistic bacteria, which could, under some conditions, cause disease. (People with weakened immune systems, infants, or elderly people may be more susceptible to infections by opportunistic microbes.) Twelve percent of the samples matched genetic sequences from pathogens that can cause disease.

In their original paper, the authors stated that two of the pathogens found in subway stations were *Yersinia pestis*, which causes bubonic plague, and *Bacillus anthracis*, the anthrax microbe, deadly bacteria that have caused widespread epidemics and suffering throughout human history. However, the interpretation of data in their publication was scrutinized and strongly criticized by the scientific community as being misleading, or even worse, sensationalistic. This forced the authors to issue a response letter and erratum (a formal correction), revising the paper and deleting their speculations about the presence of those pathogenic microbes in the subway system. The authors clarified their analysis and concluded that there is a difference between finding matching DNA fragments from a species and finding the pathogenic microbe itself.[27] Finding genetic evidence that matches segments of anthrax and plague bacterial genes does not necessarily mean that those species exist (or ever lived) in the subways, so there is no cause for panic or concern for the safety of the riders. In fact, any potential pathogens that are found in this type of survey are not likely to infect humans.[28] The survey was done by analyzing DNA, not living microbes, so traces of pathogen DNA could be from nonliving cells, remnants of organisms that lived there in the past. In addition, even if one comes into contact with disease-causing microbes, the skin, mucous, stomach acid, and immune system are typically able to ward off illness.

The scrutiny and criticism directed toward this study, and the response of the authors, illustrate how science is self-correcting. When confronted with new data and interpretations, scientists reevaluate their conclusions. If they fail to do that, the scientific community may confront the authors of a study, encouraging them to correct mistakes and change their conclusions. The website http://retractionwatch.com, which is run by the Center for Scientific Integrity, promotes the process of scrutiny and transparency in scientific inquiry and publishing. They report on retractions, corrections, and reinterpretations of scientific studies, which are important parts of the scientific process.[29]

The DNA sequencing approach used in the subway study surveys any DNA found at a site, including from living cells, dormant cells or spores, or remnants of dead organisms. Many of the microbes discovered this way may in fact be incapable of significant reproduction. In light of that, in addition to analyzing DNA to detect microbes, the subway microbiome project also looked for live organisms that could be collected and grown in the lab. Sure enough, viable bacteria that were capable of reproducing were collected from subway stations and grown on agar petri dishes. The cultured bacteria were further tested, showing that about a third of the samples were antibiotic resistant.[30] Antibiotic-resistant bacteria are of concern, as the strains that have acquired that resistance can be difficult to treat in infections. So the bottom line is, there are a lot of germs in the subways. Most of them are not harmful; however, there are microbes down there that could potentially spread disease, and since some of them are drug-resistant, they could be harder to combat in patients.

Wherever people go, they bring living germs of all sorts with them.

This published research report masterfully demonstrates the power of DNA technology to ask and answer a wide variety of fascinating questions. Not only did they get information on "who lives where in the Built Environment," but this study also provided insight into two other compelling issues.

First, in the course of this research study it was revealed that dramatic environmental changes can change the microbial life in unexpected ways. It was discovered that the South Ferry subway station, which was completely flooded during Superstorm Sandy and still remains closed, had the most unique microbiome. Ten unique species of bacteria were found there that were not seen at any of the other sites. A number of bacterial species discovered there were those that would typically be found associated with fish, in cold marine environments, such as Antarctica. The authors concluded that "the walls and floors of the station still carry a 'molecular echo' or microbiome aura of the flooding of the station with cold ocean water."[31]

The second compelling issue had to do with the discovery of animal DNA in the subway stations. The animal DNA that was found was primarily of insect origin, but there also were traces of DNA from food (chicken, meat, etc.) brought into the subways to be consumed by riders. In addition, a substantial amount of human DNA was present in every station. The investigators decided to use the human DNA to learn more about the people who use subway stations (and leave traces of themselves behind). DNA sequencing can give insight into ancestry through distinctive markers carried by different ethnic and racial groups, markers that arose during the hundreds of thousands of years of human evolution and migration across the globe. DNA sequence data, used together with programs such as Ancestry Mapper,[32] provide information on ethnic and racial background and geographic origins. By collecting and analyzing human DNA from subway stations throughout the city, it was possible to ask if ancestry clues from DNA samples are consistent with demographics of the people in the neighborhood who use the subway station. Indeed, it was possible to demonstrate that the human genetic variants found in the DNA echo the demographics of subway station neighborhoods. For instance, in a predominantly African American neighborhood, human DNA from those subway stations also had a higher representation of African genetic variants.[33] This type of comparison yielded other examples where the DNA ancestry matched the neighborhood demographics, but it was not ubiquitous, as some subway stations are in highly diverse neighborhoods or near business areas where people of many different backgrounds work.

The microecology of Superstorm Sandy and the ancestry discoveries may be tangential to the issue of hand hygiene; however, these two examples of applied DNA analysis demonstrate the power of this technology. What are some of the newfound capabilities based on DNA sequencing? We have the ability to diagnose, with great speed and accuracy, the source of deadly infections. Using DNA technology like a forensic scientist, we can determine precisely what germs are present in a particular environment ("who lives where?") and whether they pose a health risk. We have the power to detect potential threats to health from infectious agents before they cause widespread harm, whether they are of natural origin or they are due to criminal acts or bioterrorism. We can use these tools to trace the source of infectious agents, and then learn the history of their origins. As stated by Afshinnekoo and colleagues, the ability to characterize and follow changes in the microbial populations of a city "can enable a more nimble response time to any perturbations of these systems, which could potentially impact the lives of millions of people each day and billions of people each year."[34]

This conclusion to their work was not hyperbole or exaggeration of its potential impact. The microbial world is interwoven with ours and does, in fact, affect the entire human population. That is why the hospital microbiome project is a matter of life and death.

HOSPITAL MICROBIOMES

Different types of environments accumulate diverse populations of microbes. Homes, offices, and subway stations differ from each other and change over time depending on the humans, animals, and inanimate objects that pass through or set up residence; how much the areas are cleaned; and how the airflow moves the air and dust. In the nineteenth century, Ignaz Semmelweis (see chapter 2) revealed the source of infections that were killing thousands of healthy obstetrics patients a year in his Vienna hospital, and by instituting handwashing, he was able to significantly reduce the mortality rate. As we will discuss in chapter 2, it took hundreds of years for scientists and physicians to understand microbes, develop the germ theory, and learn how to combat infectious diseases, and it is still a work in progress. In modern hospitals grave health hazards still exist because of pathogenic microbes brought in by sick patients, personnel, or visitors; inadequate cleaning; and problematic HVAC systems that spread the germs. About 5 percent of patients in U.S. medical facilities (over a million people per year) develop hospital-acquired, or nosocomial, infections, which usually strike vulnerable patients from two to four days after admission and result in an estimated one hundred thousand deaths per year. It is estimated that about a third of the infections are due to lapses in hygiene protocols, that is, not washing hands or disinfecting surfaces properly.[35]

The Hospital Microbiome Project that was inaugurated in 2012 aims to better understand the problem of hospital-acquired infections. By studying the normal flora in hospital environments, it may be possible to develop strategies to enhance the benign microbes and inhibit the disease-causing ones. The University of Chicago Medical Center was constructing a new hospital pavilion in 2012, and they wished to monitor the evolution of the microbial environment as the clinics and wards started being populated by patients. Basic principles of the proposed study included the notion that beneficial microbes could inhibit or crowd out pathogens, that patients with germs are the source of infections that spread, and that areas dedicated to patient care would be the most common source of infectious agents. The Alfred P. Sloan Foundation provided $850,000 in funding for surveying the microbiome before, during, and after patients arrived in the new wards.[36]

Jack Gilbert, one of the lead scientists involved in this initiative, maintains that "the kill-all approach isn't working."[37] In other words, if it were possible to introduce harmless commensal bacteria to hospital surfaces, perhaps it would crowd out the pathogenic species. The idea is that a truly sterile environment is difficult to establish and impossible to maintain, so why bother? Maybe it would be better to flood the environment with friendly microbes. The ongoing study is hoping to figure out how the populations of microbes fluctuate over time, in order to devise strategies to reduce the spread of the dangerous inhabitants.

Preliminary data suggest that the situation is incredibly complex and dynamic, with changes in the microbiome of a hospital room seen within a few hours. HVAC systems are of major concern, and redesign of the heating, ventilation, and air-conditioning ducts could reduce cross-contamination between hospital rooms and spaces. But all agree that behavioral changes and improvement in basic hygienic procedures would make an enormous difference in reducing the risks to patients. "Hand washing—key to controlling the spread of many diseases—remains inadequate among hospital staff despite numerous educational campaigns."[38] Hand hygiene in hospitals will be explored in depth in chapter 3.

The Failure to Wash Hands

Despite the billions of dollars we spend on soap, body wash, shampoo, toothpaste, mouthwash, and so on, we do not always accomplish what is necessary to keep us healthy. Studies have shown that a surprising percentage of Americans do not wash their hands after using the toilet. We pride ourselves on teaching children hygiene, and schools have numerous programs to teach handwashing techniques. Almost all the books published about handwashing are directed at children. But something happens when Americans grow up—or when their mothers aren't watching. They stop washing their hands! There is also a discrepancy between the practices of the sexes: women are more likely to wash (but still far from perfect in washing their hands when needed). There are differences between hygienic practices at different ages and life stages. We have a long way to go to practice what we preach.

The hand microbiome was surveyed in fifty-one healthy college students from the University of Colorado, finding on average more than 150 "distinct species-level bacterial phylotypes" on each palm surface.[39] This is three times the diversity of microbes found on the forearm or elbow, and equivalent to, or possibly more diverse than, the microbes found in the gut or mouth. It is not shocking that the hand, which touches so many diverse surfaces, picks up so many different microbes. What is surprising is that there is immense variation between the phylotypes found on different people's hands. Out of a total of 4,742 unique phylotypes that were identified across all 102 palms that were tested, only five of those phylotypes were common to all the hands. The left hand and the right hand of the same person were also significantly different, typically sharing only 17 percent of the microbe phylotypes. Comparing one person to another, an average of 13 percent of species were the same (with the other 87 percent being unique).[40]

Men and women harbor significantly different populations of microbes, with women demonstrating more diversity in the phyla found on their hands. The authors speculate on possible explanations for the differences between male and female hands, including differences in skin pH (men's skin is more acidic), hormones, sweat, sebum, use of hand creams or cosmetics, and/or handwashing frequency.[41]

Another significant factor in the microbiome composition was the time that had elapsed since the last handwashing, and since women report more frequent handwashing than men, it might influence the distribution of bacteria on their hands. Curious about this, the researchers conducted a smaller study of eight people, four men and four women. They had the volunteers wash their hands, and then their palms were swabbed every two hours for a six-hour period. That study confirmed that even when handwashing is controlled and identical in men and women, the two genders still differ significantly in hand microbiomes. In addition, over several hours the microbial population on palms changes significantly, with women ending up with a greater diversity of phylotypes than men. This study showed that handwashing frequency may not be the major contributor to observed differences in men's and women's palms. It also demonstrated that hands repopulate with bacteria soon after washing.[42]

That being said, who is washing hands, and how often? Handwashing is a frequent topic at the annual meeting of the ASM, the American Society for Microbiology. At the 2003 meeting of that group, a report on hand hygiene in airport bathrooms in six major cities showed that more people wash their hands in the Toronto airport after using the toilet (more than 95 percent) than in Miami (81 percent), Chicago's O'Hare (73 percent), or New York's JFK (70 percent). The overall rate for all subjects was 78 percent, which was an improvement from the 68 percent rate found in 1996 and 2000. Females outperformed males in Toronto, Dallas/Fort Worth, Miami, O'Hare, and JFK. The only exception to this was at San Francisco International, where 80 percent of men were observed to wash, compared with less than 60 percent of women.[43] That may be the only documented example of men outperforming women in handwashing. San Francisco is clearly a unique city in many ways.

At the ASM meeting in 2010, investigators reported on a study done at Turner Field, home of the Atlanta Braves, which showed a mere two-thirds of men washing their hands in public restrooms, compared to an impressive 98 percent of women who were observed to wash.[44] This is entirely speculation, but perhaps some men felt a need to rush back to the game, while women had other motivations (such as trying to wash off germs acquired from sitting in a dirty stadium?). Other revelations at that ASM meeting were that 20 percent of people using the bathrooms at Grand Central Station and Pennsylvania Station in Manhattan did not wash their hands.[45] Those people go from bathroom usage back into the stations and into subway cars, where they can spread whatever germs they have acquired on their hands.

In contrast with the observed behaviors, when polled in a phone survey 96 percent of people claim to wash their hands after using public washrooms, and 89 percent claim to wash up at home.[46] Clearly there is a discrepancy between the self-reported and observed behaviors; perhaps because of peer pressure and embarrassment, many more people claim to wash than actually do it. Since handwashing is socially desirable, it would follow that people will lie about their habits. The numbers of people who do wash up was higher in 2010 than in previous years, possibly because of the H1N1 influenza pandemic that made people more aware of the risk of infection.[47]

While we teach our children well when they are small, when they are out of sight, on their own, what do they do? Many middle- and high-school-age children do not have a very good record of handwashing after using the bathroom. In a study of children from two single-sex private schools in Pennsylvania, 120 students were observed, once again confirming that females have significantly higher rates of handwashing than males. Fifty-eight percent of girls washed their hands after using the bathroom compared with 48 percent of boys. Only 28 percent of girls and 8 percent of boys used soap, and females washed for more than five seconds 50 percent of the time, compared with 23 percent of male students who exceeded five seconds of washing.[48] Clearly we need to do a better job teaching basic hygiene from the very beginning. Of course, the teen years are a time of pushing boundaries and taking chances; perhaps college students do better.

Many college students live away from home for the first time in their lives and are making their own decisions. Research on college students living in a university dormitory revealed that females once again outdid males in hand hygiene. Sixty-nine percent of females wash after urinating compared with 43 percent of males, and 84 percent of females wash their hands after defecation, compared with 78 percent of males. A very small percentage of students report that they always wash before eating: only 10 percent of males and 7 percent of females.[49] This is an important statistic, since the transmission of infections is frequently from hand or other surfaces to mouth. We do not emphasize handwashing with regard to food consumption, or before eating, nearly enough.

In another college-related study, three scientists from the School of Hospitality Business at Michigan State University studied "Hand Washing Practices in a College Town Environment," hoping to learn more about the demographics of handwashing, whether washroom environments may influence handwashing, and whether people are really washing well enough. The fact is that many people wash (actually rinse) without soap and believe that is adequate. This project defined three categories of hand hygiene after use of the toilet: (1) no washing at all, (2) washing without soap, which the authors refer to as "attempted washing," and (3) washing hands with soap. They classified the 3,749 subjects into two age groups: college age or younger, and older than college age. The study found that 66.9 percent of subjects washed with soap; 23 percent washed with water alone, and 10.3 percent did not wash their hands at all after using the toilet. The gender gap once again was confirmed, with 77.9 percent of women washing with soap compared to 50.3 percent of men. The nonwasher group included 7 percent of the women and 14.6 percent of the men. And subjects in the older group washed hands with soap 70.3 percent of the time compared with 64.8 percent of younger subjects. All differences observed were statistically significant.[50]

The study also revealed that when there were signs posted in the bathroom encouraging handwashing, people were more likely to use soap. Also, when the sinks were clean (vs. "reasonably clean" or dirty) subjects were more likely to wash with soap, but the faucet type (standard vs. motion detection) had no effect on handwashing behavior. Those results suggest that while some environmental conditions could affect hand hygiene, others are not so important. Whether or not the faucet turns itself on did not appear to make a difference. But posting a sign to remind people to wash their hands, or keeping the sink clean, could significantly improve handwashing behavior.[51]

Effectiveness of Handwashing to Reduce Risk of Infectious Diseases

At last we get to the crux of the matter. There is much evidence that hands can serve as vectors for the transmission of disease. Chapter 2 further discusses the scientific discoveries related to how hands serve as reservoirs of germs that cause infection and illness. And we have just learned that many people fail to wash their hands even after using the toilet or before eating. There are so many wrong ways to practice hand hygiene. What actually works?

Shigella are bacteria that infect the gut, causing diarrhea, cramps, nausea, vomiting, and sometimes fever or more severe symptoms. Shigellosis is highly contagious and can continue for months within a community, being transmitted from person to person. The most effective approach to reduce the risk of catching it is handwashing. One *Shigella* outbreak in North Texas schools was reported in a 2012 article entitled, "How We Didn't Clean Up until We Washed Our Hands: Shigellosis in an Elementary and Middle School in North Texas." After a number of cases arose, doctors, hospitals, and schools were canvassed to figure out where it had started. The disease was traced back to the index case, that is, the first person who got it, a music teacher at the schools. That teacher most likely had transmitted the disease to some students, who passed it on to others, to the point where 10 percent of the student body was sick, and other family members in fifteen families had caught it. This bacteria could have gone on to infect many more, but healthcare personnel reacted by installing liquid soap dispensers in washrooms, and providing students and staff with instruction and prompting on how and when to wash hands. They scheduled handwashing times into the day, and they implemented cleaning and disinfection protocols for materials in the schools that are commonly handled. These steps stopped the outbreak, and no new cases arose.[52]

In addition to the North Texas case, there have been hundreds of other

studies that support the role of handwashing in reducing infectious disease. One effective way to compare and assess research done on different
populations is by meta-analysis. Statisticians and epidemiologists are able
to look at a variety of research projects that vary in sample size, methodology, and rigor to determine which ones are more meaningful, which
are comparable, whether the different studies contradict each other, or
whether taken together they can provide stronger evidence to support
correlation or causative effects. For instance, the idea that handwashing
reduces the risk of diarrhea was studied by meta-analysis of seventeen separate studies on disease and hand hygiene. By considering the results of
these studies (on varied populations, in different parts of the world, with
different diseases) the analysis concludes that handwashing can reduce
the risk of diarrhea by up to 47 percent. Taking into account the populations that are at risk, the authors suggest that "interventions to promote
handwashing might save a million lives."[53] This puts handwashing into
perspective. It's not just about the sniffles; it is about multitudes of people
suffering from disease and death.

Another meta-analysis identified thirty studies from 1960 through
2007. By comparing and combining results they found that improving
handwashing reduced the rates of gastrointestinal illnesses by 31 percent
and of respiratory illnesses by 21 percent. Hand hygiene with traditional
soap worked the best, and antibacterial soap added little if any benefit to
the reduction in disease.[54]

Another meta-analysis was performed on sixteen research studies conducted in schools, households, child-care centers, elderly daycare, offices,
and low-income squatter settlements. These studies all addressed hand-
hygiene interventions and respiratory infections, including influenza.
Despite the great diversity of settings, populations, and communities,
handwashing interventions were associated with reduction in infections
of the respiratory tract and influenza risk. In the various studies included
in the meta-analysis, the relationship between disease and handwashing
ranged from modest to more dramatic, depending on many factors. For
instance, in the study of impoverished people who were living as squatters,
hand-hygiene intervention was highly effective at reducing infections. In
other cases there was some improvement, but it was not as significant.[55]
But the fact that teaching, training, and modeling handwashing works in

so many different situations and communities supports the notion that it is worthwhile to improve handwashing at any level.

Handwashing Agents

SOAP AND WATER VERSUS WATER ALONE

As described previously, many research studies on handwashing show that while many people use soap and water to wash, a large proportion of the population wash their hands with water alone after using the bathroom. Does washing with water alone reduce contamination? What are the best agents to reduce contamination on hands, and to reduce the risk of infectious disease?

A British study found that washing with water alone does reduce germs. The British research team sent twenty volunteers out to contaminate their hands by touching surfaces in a busy British museum, on public buses, and in the Underground. When they returned to the lab, they were assigned to (1) wash their hands using soap and water, (2) wash their hands using water alone, or (3) not wash at all. Each volunteer did this 24 times, that is, 8 times for each of the hand treatments (480 total conditions for the 20 volunteers). Bacterial contaminants were analyzed, showing that the subjects brought back a variety of microbes that they had picked up by touching public surfaces. Bacterial contamination was found on 44 percent of the hands that were not washed, on 23 percent of the hands washed with water alone, and on 8 percent of the hands washed with soap and water. So washing with water alone helps to decontaminate hands significantly, but it is not as effective as washing with soap and water.[56]

In Bangladesh people are living in conditions that those of us in more developed countries would find hard to relate to. There are high levels of child mortality that could be reduced by simple hygienic practices. Handwashing seems to be a simple remedy that anyone could adopt. But for people living in subsistence conditions even fresh water is a luxury, and soap may be unaffordable. A fascinating study surveyed handwashing behavior in Bangladeshi homes that had no hygiene interventions, to determine if there was a relationship between even the most rudimentary approaches to handwashing and child diarrhea. Three hundred and forty-seven households in fifty rural villages were studied over the course of two years. Compared to homes where the food preparer did not wash their hands at all, diarrhea was reduced in homes where food was prepared after washing at least one hand with water alone. The risk was further reduced when both hands were washed with water, or at least one hand was washed with soap.[57] Washing with water alone is better than not washing at all.

But washing with soap is better still. "Hand Washing with Soap: The Most Effective 'Do-It-Yourself' Vaccine?" is a review article written by researchers from Pune, India. While Pune is a growing and developing metropolis east of Mumbai, a large proportion of its population still resides in slums with rudimentary hygiene. The authors strongly endorse handwashing, noting that "hand washing with soap . . . may be more effective than any single vaccine or hygiene behaviour. Promoted broadly enough, hand washing with soap can be viewed as an essential do-it-yourself vaccine." The washing procedure described in that paper is derived from a variety of sources. Use of water alone is not sufficient, as the skin is covered with oils and fats that do not dissolve in water and could trap bacteria. Soaps and detergents dissolve oils and that helps to release contaminants from the skin. The authors discuss solid soap bars, explaining that since the bars are reused they could transfer bacteria from person to person. They recommend washing the soap bar off before and after use. Plain soap is recommended, as it has the same effectiveness as antibacterial soap in terms of washing microbes off the skin. Soap and warm running water produce the best cleansing conditions. The recommended approach is: First, make a lather from soap and water that is rubbed on all surfaces of the hands (including under the nails) for a minimum of twenty seconds. Then the hands should be rinsed under warm running water and dried with a clean cloth towel or paper towel. The drying step also helps to remove contaminants. The authors cited a study that found that the use of warm-air hand dryers can increase bacteria on the hands, while paper towels further reduce the bacteria on hands. (See later in this chapter for more on hand drying.) They also addressed medical handwashing, which will be discussed in chapter 3.[58]

ANTIBACTERIAL SOAPS

There is a huge controversy with regard to antibacterial soaps, but this is not a new story. In the 1950s an antibacterial chemical called hexachlorophene was invented and used in skin cleansers such as pHisohex and

Dial soap. Many teenagers used pHisohex since its antibacterial properties were effective against acne. It also was used in clinical settings as a disinfectant. However, it turns out that hexachlorophene is very toxic, and in 1972 the FDA discontinued its use in many products.

Hexachlorophene was replaced in some products with triclosan. For many years it has been one of the ingredients in toothpaste (Colgate's Total toothpaste has had it since 1997, as it reduces the incidence of gingivitis), hand soap, and many other products for human use, but now it is under suspicion of being hazardous to health. The molecular structures of hexachlorophene and triclosan have similar shapes. They both are organic chemicals, with two phenol (six carbon) rings and chlorine atoms. (Hexachlorophene has six chlorine atoms per molecule; triclosan has three chlorines, hence its name. There are several dozen trade names that are synonyms for triclosan, and some examples are Ultra-Fresh, Microban, and Biofresh.) The FDA began to suspect problems with triclosan forty years ago when it first appeared, but failed to pursue the issue. The FDA, while permitting its use, never classified triclosan as "generally recognized as safe and effective," that is, GRAS/GRAE, a status conferred only on chemicals that have been established as safe and effective in a series of research studies. Triclosan was given the FDA classification IIISE, with status III meaning additional data are needed, S indicating safety data and E indicating effectiveness data. There was not enough scientific research available for the FDA to confer GRAS/GRAE status on triclosan back in the 1970s, and that situation never changed.[59]

In the last two decades there has been a trend of increased interest in antibacterial consumer goods, and the use of triclosan spread; it was introduced into products as diverse as socks and lunch boxes.[60] Meanwhile, over time research on triclosan turned up some very disturbing revelations. The chemical is absorbed by our skin or mucus membranes and is found in 97 percent of breast milk samples and in human blood plasma. It passes through our bodies and is found in the urine of 75 percent of people tested.[61] Triclosan may affect levels of reproductive hormones, such as testosterone and estrogen, and in female rats it can lead to early puberty.[62] One concern has been that the use of antibacterials such as triclosan can lead to the development of antibiotic-resistant strains of bacteria, the so-called "superbugs" that are killing patients as drug-resistant diseases become more and more difficult to treat.[63] And triclosan is reportedly found in 60 percent of U.S. streams and rivers tested and in agricultural soil.[64] The most recent alarm is that triclosan has been shown to be a tumor promoter, which means that under certain circumstances it can stimulate mouse liver cell growth, possibly pushing precancerous cells to become carcinoma cells.[65]

The disturbing findings led the FDA to launch an in-depth review of the mounting data against triclosan and finally declare in 2013 that "based on the currently available data, this proposed rule finds that consumer antiseptic wash active ingredients can be considered neither safe nor effective for use in OTC [over the counter] consumer antiseptic wash drug products." The FDA report recommends manufacturer's compliance — removal of triclosan — within a year of "a final rule."[66] The final rule has not yet been implemented, so federal regulations on triclosan are still up in the air. Meanwhile, Minnesota became the first state to ban triclosan from consumer hygiene products in May 2014, a ban that will take effect on January 1, 2017.[67]

In light of the mounting evidence that triclosan may be hazardous to human health and the environment, the bad press surrounding it, and current and pending legislation, some manufacturers have responded by voluntarily removing triclosan from their products. Crest toothpaste is now proudly triclosan-free. In addition, the European Union put restrictions on its use, and the Kaiser Permanente medical system (thirty-seven hospitals across the United States) has become triclosan-free.

The FDA also found insufficient evidence of *any* benefit in washing with triclosan-containing soaps compared to traditional soaps.[68] The bottom line is, washing with soap and water is tried and true and a highly effective approach to hygiene; no triclosan is needed or desired.

ASHES, ASHES, WE ALL FALL DOWN

In addition to the traditional soap and water that Americans are accustomed to, there are other approaches to keeping hands clean that are more unconventional. In some parts of the world water is at a premium, and soap may be difficult to find or prohibitively expensive. Thus, in rural parts of India and Bangladesh, ash and mud are sometimes used as cleansing agents. Researchers studied forty households with small children in

Rajendranagar, Andhra Pradesh, India to determine if washing hands with ash was effective in reducing bacterial contamination. Hand contamination was reduced significantly with the use of ash or soap as a cleanser.[69]

Another study confirmed the usefulness of traditional Bangladeshi hand hygiene. Twenty women living in a slum of Dhaka, Bangladesh, were asked to wash their hands on different occasions with ash, soap, mud, and plain water. The women lived in a community in bamboo huts with earthen floors. In that community, soap is rarely used because it is costly; and in that society, after defecation most people typically cleanse their left hands only by rubbing them on the ground and rinsing with water. In this experiment the ash and mud were presterilized, and the water was obtained from a clean well. Hands were tested for the presence of fecal coliform bacteria under varied conditions. With no washing, 60 percent (12/20) of the hands were fecal coliform positive; after washing with water alone, 40 percent (8/20) of the hands were positive, which was not a statistically significant difference. After washing with soap or mud, the figure dropped to 20 percent (4/20), and with ash to 15 percent (3/20) of hands fecal testing as coliform positive. The reduction in contamination using soap, ash, or mud was statistically significant, but the three agents were not significantly different from each other. This shows that under these conditions, in rural Bangladesh where women use rudimentary approaches for hand hygiene, ash, mud, or soap have similar efficacy, and any of these three approaches is better than not washing or using water alone.[70] While the use of ash or mud is a significant improvement over no washing at all, it is still a long way from establishing a healthy environment. When hands are contaminated 15 or 20 percent of the time, there is significant risk of disease transmission.

Ash, mud, and soil may be convenient, available, and cheap in developing countries, and they do have some value in reducing hand contamination, but those three agents are also potentially contaminated themselves. Pathogens can thrive in soil and mud; in particular, bacteria, viruses, protozoa, and parasitic worms are known to reside actively or lie dormant for long periods of time in those environments. In developing countries many people do not have toilets or any plumbing, and they defecate in the soil, possibly near a river or stream that can overflow and sweep the waste to other areas. Animal waste also accumulates around the living areas and can contaminate soil or mud or even the ashes from the household fire. Under those conditions, washing with ash or mud or soil could increase the risk of infection, rather than decrease it. In addition, local pollutants can contaminate the soil; these could include pesticides or toxic heavy metals such as lead, chromium, or arsenic, which can sicken or kill people who are exposed to them.[71] Therefore, unless there is no other alternative, wash up with soap and water, not with ash, mud, or soil.

ALCOHOL RUBS

Waterless hand sanitizers have become popular, as they provide a way to reduce hand contamination in the absence of water. Most of these products are alcohol based, and they come in convenient dispensers of all sizes and shapes: pocket-size tubes, pumps, automatic dispensers, wall-mounted devices, handy wipes, and even miniature vials that dangle from your neck or keychain. They are particularly useful when a sink and running water is not conveniently available.

There are an estimated three billion people on our planet who do not have clean running water conveniently available.[72] They live without plumbing, some without access to wells, and many have to travel, often by foot, to get the day's supply of drinking and cooking water, with little to spare for hygiene. But in order to reduce the spread of infectious diseases in those communities, hand hygiene is of paramount importance. One possible solution? Alcohol-based hand sanitizers. A research study was done comparing the effectiveness of handwashing with soap to using alcohol-based hand sanitizers in a community in Dar es Salaam, Tanzania, a region with limited access to clean running water. The goal of the project was to determine whether the availability of waterless hand sanitizers could provide better access and improve hand hygiene with the hope of reducing disease in such environments.[73]

The results were not very impressive in terms of reducing microbes on hands. The subjects, who were local mothers, cleansed their hands with either hand sanitizer or soap and water. The presence of *E. coli* and fecal *Streptococci* are good indicators of contamination with feces. When we measure bacteria, we calculate their growth by culturing them in the millions or billions, so we use logarithms, or powers of ten, to express relative amounts of cells. Keeping in mind that each logarithmic unit is a tenfold change, with the starting number of bacteria set at 100 percent, a 1.0 log unit reduction leaves 10 percent of the bacteria, and a 2.0 log unit reduction leaves a mere 1 percent of the bacteria.

Use of hand sanitizer resulted in an average of 0.66 log reductions per hand for *E. coli* bacteria, compared with 0.50 log reductions with soap and water, not a statistically significant difference. Hand sanitizer reduced fecal *Streptococci* by 0.64 log units per hand, compared with soap and water, which only reduced it by 0.25 log units; this was a statistically significant difference in effectiveness.[74] The outcomes of the hand-hygiene trials in this study were not very impressive with regard to cleansing. Recall that a 1.0 log reduction means that bacteria have been reduced by 90 percent. This sounds pretty useful, but it still leaves 10 percent of the microbes that you would find on an unwashed hand. Log reduction values found in the study were less than 1.0, namely 0.66, 0.64, 0.50, and 0.25, representing much less than a 90 percent reduction in each instance, which are not very impressive reductions in hand contamination, leaving lots of bacteria still on the hands. Despite the fact that the subjects did not cleanse their hands all that well, the goals of the research study are worthy, as they are hoping to learn how to improve hand hygiene in challenging environments.

The same research team had better results a year later when they tested alcohol-based hand sanitizer (ABHS) on soiled, dirty hands. Hands that were visibly soiled with Tanzanian dirt or with cooking oil were deliberately contaminated with *E. coli* bacteria. Upon treatment with hand sanitizer, the cleansing achieved a reduction of more than 2 log units, in other words, a more than 99 percent reduction in bacteria, suggesting that alcohol rub can be a useful cleanser.[75]

Yet another study, this time in Canada, found that soap and water is more effective than alcohol-based hand sanitizers or antiseptic hand wipes. The ten volunteer subjects in this research project had their hands contaminated with a nontoxigenic strain of *Clostridium difficile*.[76] The toxigenic form of the bacteria is notorious for causing hospital-acquired infections that are very difficult to eradicate. Of course, no one would want to expose subjects to the disease-causing form; the nontoxigenic strain they used for the study is much safer since it does not produce the toxins that disrupt the gut, resulting in life-threatening disease symptoms.

The hand cleansing in this study was fairly successful. Warm water and soap reduced bacteria by an average of 2.14 log units (leaving less than 1 percent of the original bacteria). Cold water and soap reduced the contamination by 1.88 log units; warm water and antibacterial soap reduced it by 1.51 log units; antiseptic hand wipes by 0.57 log units; and alcohol-based hand rub by 0.06 log units. The last condition, the alcohol rub, was statistically no more effective than not washing at all. The authors conclude the paper by strongly recommending handwashing with soap and water, rather than using alcohol-based hand rubs, when faced with *C. difficile* infections.[77] Other studies have confirmed that *C. difficile* is not eliminated with alcohol-based hand rub. So the choice of handwashing agent will differ depending on the bacteria of concern, with one study concluding, "Residual [*C. Difficile*] spores are readily transferred by a handshake after use of ABHR [alcohol-based hand rub]."[78] *C. difficile* is generally not a threat to healthy people; it is more likely to occur in hospital populations or in patients who are taking antibiotics that disrupt the gut microbiome, enabling the *C. difficile* strain to dominate. Many other disease-causing germs are eliminated by alcohol treatment.

The most important outcome of hand cleansing is on the actual health of people. Do individuals who use alcohol-based hand sanitizers avoid getting sick? Are there lower rates of transmission of infectious disease in environments where hand sanitizers are used? The answer is a resounding "yes"! Alcohol-based hand gels reduce the transmission of illnesses in elementary schools and absenteeism among the students.[79] And an increase in hand-hygiene behavior, including the use of alcohol-based hand gels, reduces the incidence of illness and absenteeism in college students who live in residence halls. In one study, the test group had 43 percent fewer missed school or workdays.[80] Alcohol-based hand gels also reduce the transmission of respiratory illnesses in the home.[81] That is noteworthy, since that is how many of us contract illnesses—from our sick children, our spouses or significant others, and other family members. Our home is where we live in close proximity with our loved ones, touching the same surfaces and each other; sharing spaces intimately; picking up the same phones, utensils, dishes, and towels; and using the same toilets, sinks, and bathing areas.

One explanation for the frequent transmission of germs throughout the household is that there is still widespread ignorance about how infectious diseases spread. In one study of families with children in daycare,

researchers were surprised to learn that only 66 percent of parents correctly believed that colds could be transmitted by direct contact, such as
shaking hands with a sick person, and fewer than half believed that to be
true about stomach flus. Only 43 percent knew that eating food prepared
by a sick person can increase the risk of transmission of stomach flu, and
only 35 percent understood that changing the diapers of a sick child could
lead to transmission of disease, through fecal-oral transmission. There is
a serious disconnect between the advances in scientific understanding of
microbiology and the general public's use of that knowledge. For instance,
33 percent said that they always wash their hands after blowing or wiping a
nose, 72 percent claim to always wash after changing a diaper, and 84 percent after using the bathroom. That leaves a lot of people with germ-laden
hands. That study revealed that homes with small children in daycare
have high rates of transmission of respiratory and gastrointestinal illness,
which is not a great surprise to anyone who has ever had children in day-
care. The good news is that the use of alcohol-based hand gel was associated with reduced transmission of secondary respiratory infections. The
bad news is that only about 8 percent of respondents use alcohol-based
hand rub all or most of the time at home. The authors suggest that educational interventions are called for, as there is a need to better inform people about how germs are spread and the options for eradicating them.[82]

How to Wash Hands

Handwashing: We have all been doing it since we were old enough for our
mothers to bring or carry us to the sink and guide our grimy little hands
under the running water. There have been entire books written on the subject (and you are reading one of them). But it's not only about "rinse, lather
with soap for a count of twenty, rinse again." It is about the culture, the
science, and the motivation to actually do it well. To demonstrate the importance of hand hygiene, there is a comprehensive tome on the science of
hand hygiene that is a 262-page manual (8.5-by-11-inch, double-column,
7-point font) called WHO *Guidelines on Hand Hygiene in Healthcare: First
Global Patient Safety Challenge/Clean Care Is Safer Care*.[83] This manual,
which cites 1,168 scientific references, presents everything you would ever
want to know about washing and cleansing hands for the clinical setting.

The information also is relevant to hygiene practices in schools, institutions, and the home, as for the most part the same principles apply—after all, germs are germs, wherever they are. The manual has chapters on skin, bacteria, transmission, hand-rub and handwashing agents, technique, economic impact, and many more topics. It is written for healthcare professionals who have compelling reasons to master this skill. (In chapter 3 we will discuss how some healthcare professionals fail to comply with protocols on hand hygiene, and what we can do about it.)

Here is the technique for hand hygiene, as described by the WHO manual:

Alcohol-based hand rub: "Apply a palmful of alcohol-based hand rub and cover all surfaces of the hands. Rub hands until dry."[84]

Soap and water: "When washing hands with soap and water, wet hands with water and apply the amount of product [liquid, bar, leaf, or powdered soap] necessary to cover all surfaces. Rinse hands with water and dry thoroughly with a single-use towel. Use clean, running water whenever possible. Avoid using hot water, as repeated exposure to hot water may increase risk of dermatitis. Use towel to turn off tap/faucet. Dry hands thoroughly using a method that does not recontaminate hands."[85]

That's it. The rest, as they say, is commentary. For instance, how long should the hands be scrubbed with soap? There is a consensus that soaping up should last a minimum of fifteen to twenty seconds, or about the time it takes to sing the "Happy Birthday Song" twice. Of course, surgical handwashing is more complicated (see chapter 3), but even that is not rocket science.

As to what type or form of soap to use, there are many, many choices of fine and effective soaps. We have just learned that the so-called "antibacterial" soaps do not add much, if anything, to the efficacy of washing. Bar soap may not be the best choice in places where many people use the facilities because the bars are sitting in open, moist vessels and can accumulate germs from one person that get passed on to another.

Best practices in hand hygiene in child-care facilities are described in *Caring for Our Children: National Health and Safety Performance Standards: Guidelines for Early Care and Early Education Programs*, published under the auspices of the American Academy of Pediatrics, the American Public Health Association, and the National Resource Center for Health and

Safety in Child Care and Early Education.[86] Among the standards specified in the document, the American Academy of Pediatrics (AAP) and the other two august groups recommend that handwashing be performed by staff and children with dispensed liquid soap and running water. They do not recommend bar soaps or antibacterial soaps, neither do they recommend premoistened cleansing towelettes, as they are not effective for cleaning hands. If necessary when there is no access to running water, the use of an alcohol-based hand sanitizer is acceptable. Alcohol-based hand sanitizer is not suitable for children younger than two years old.

The guidelines describe how to assist young children with the task and recommend that after helping a child to wash, the staff member needs to wash his or her own hands. Guidelines for teaching children and for training staff are included. These steps should be followed:[87]

1 Check to be sure a clean, disposable paper (or single-use cloth) towel is available.
2 Turn on warm water, between 60 degrees F. and 120 degrees F., to a comfortable temperature.
3 Moisten hands with water and apply soap (not antibacterial) to hands.
4 Rub hands together vigorously until a soapy lather appears, hands are out of the water stream, and continue for at least twenty seconds (sing "Happy Birthday" silently twice). Rub areas between fingers, around nail beds, under fingernails, jewelry, and back of hands. Nails should be kept short; acrylic nails should not be worn.
5 Rinse hands under running water, between 60 degrees F. and 120 degrees F., until they are free of soap and dirt. Leave the water running while drying hands.
6 Dry hands with the clean, disposable paper or single-use cloth towel.
7 If taps do not shut off automatically, turn taps off with a disposable paper or single-use cloth towel.
8 Throw the disposable paper towel into a lined trash container; or place single-use cloth towels in the laundry hamper; or hang individually labeled cloth towels to dry. Use hand lotion to prevent chapping of hands, if desired.

Note that a wide temperature range is recommended, as water ranging from cool (60 degrees F.) to warm (120 degrees F.) is effective for cleansing with soap. Hot water is not recommended as it can dry out the skin more, leading to chapped hands and abrasions. Some other recommendations include when to wash hands during the day, that is, all staff and children should wash upon arrival at the facility, and before and after handling food or feeding a child, treating a skin ailment or wound, diapering, or giving medication. In addition, they should wash hands after handling garbage, after using the bathroom or assisting a child in the bathroom, after handling any bodily fluids (vomit, blood, or mucus), after handling animals, and after outdoor play, especially in sandboxes. If staff members go (preferably off premises) to smoke, they should wash their hands when they return to prevent exposing children to thirdhand smoke.

The Golden Rule of hygiene is that hands should be cleansed with running water and dispensed soap, at appropriate times, and when in doubt, wash your hands.

Hand Drying

Lest you think that's the end of the story, think again. The very act of drying hands is rife with potential problems, problems of the recontamination of hands. You do not want to undo the good of handwashing in the process of drying hands.

First of all, hand drying is very important as wet surfaces readily harbor, sustain, and transmit germs more effectively than dry surfaces. Microbes love moisture. Keeping hands dry and minimizing the touching of wet surfaces goes a long way toward reducing the transmission of germs. The main choices for hand drying are cloth towels, paper towels (of different kinds), warm-air dryers, and jet-air dryers. Cloth towels are typically used at home, and each person in the household should have their own towel and space to hang it. There are people who will use a bath towel only once before laundering. If not shared, it is reasonable to reuse one's personal cloth towel as long as it is permitted to dry between uses and laundered on a regular basis. Meaghan Murphy of *Good Housekeeping* magazine recommends that people can use bath towels to dry off after a shower up to three times before laundering, but suggests changing frequently used hand towels more often, perhaps every day or two.[88] Paper towels are disposable and single use, so there is no issue of shared germs. But they can be pricey and the waste adds up, contributing to environmental waste disposal issues. Some people provide paper towels for guests in the home, or use them in the kitchen for cleanup.

In public washrooms the drying possibilities provided are generally paper, warm-air, or jet-air dryers. In very old-fashioned washrooms, it is possible to still find the reusable cloth roller towels with which each user can unroll a fresh segment of cloth as needed. The soiled, used part gets wound up back inside the unit and is presumably taken out and laundered and replaced with a fresh roll. When the end of the roll is reached, no fresh segments can be exposed, and this is an issue, as numerous users can end up repeatedly using the same section. I never had much faith in cloth roller towels, and I recall my father cautioning us about it, as he did not trust the cleanliness of this system. This system is all but extinct, so it does not warrant further analysis. (If you encounter this on your travels back in time, or when you go to some remote regions or foreign countries, you may have to make the choice of using it or walking away with wet hands. On a recent trip to Africa, I encountered this cloth roller system and chose the latter—allowing my wet hands to air dry.)

A few years ago a decision was made to remove paper towels from many of the restrooms at my university and replace them with warm-air dryers. This move was done to save money on paper towels and reduce waste in the environment. I never had much tolerance for warm-air dryers, as I do not have the patience to stand and wait up to a minute for the air stream to thoroughly dry my hands. I don't much care for the noise either. I was not too happy about this change, as I dislike damp hands or touching restroom doorknobs. So I got into the habit of bringing a few paper towels with me to the bathroom, to dry my hands and open the door to leave. It turns out that without conducting any formal research project beyond my own experience, I was on target in terms of my suspicion and dislike of warm-air dryers. Paper towels are far superior to warm-air dryers for drying, as well as for reducing microbes and the transmission of microbes. Paper towels also beat out jet dryers for reducing microbes and transmission of microbes.

The good news is that when our new science building was built, the restrooms were equipped with jet dryers as well as automatic (touchless) paper towel dispensers. When there is a choice of hand drying methods to use, it is useful to know which method is safest in terms of hand hygiene.

A comprehensive study comparing paper towels, warm-air dryers, and jet-air dryers was conducted by Keith Redway and Shameem Fawdar of the University of Westminster, London.[89] The study was prepared for the European Tissue Symposium, which is sponsored by the European Tissue Paper Industry Association, so there may be conflict-of-interest issues with regard to this study. In addition, this study does not appear to have been published in a peer-reviewed journal. Nevertheless, the project appears to be well designed with regard to research protocol, and the data appear to be analyzed properly as well.

The first part of the project compared the drying efficiency of five different types of paper towels, a warm-air dryer, and a jet-air dryer. How fast do the three approaches actually dry hands? To determine the dryness of hands, the researchers measured the amount of water removed by weighing paper towels before and after drying hands and subtracting the difference. The percentage of dryness was calculated using the difference between fully wet hands and hands that have gone through a drying process using a particular drying method.[90] Hand dryness was monitored for seven methods (five types of paper towels, a warm-air dryer, and a jet-air dryer) at ten-second intervals over sixty seconds. The five types of paper towels were very similar to each other with regard to speed of drying. Four out of five of them achieved more than 90 percent dryness within 10 seconds (one type took 20 seconds to exceed 90 percent dryness). The jet-air dryer was also very efficient and achieved 89.3 percent dryness within 10 seconds. However, the warm-air dryer only achieved about 34 percent dryness by 10 seconds, 55 percent by 20 seconds, 71 percent by 30 seconds, 84 percent by 40 seconds, and 92 percent by 50 seconds.[91] Do you know anyone willing to stand in a public restroom for almost a minute drying their hands thoroughly in a warm-air dryer? I would never do that, and neither would most other people, as the same research study showed the average time spent drying with warm-air dryers is approximately 20 seconds. Recall that wet hands conduct and transmit germs more readily than dry ones do, and combine that with the notion that most people who walk away from warm-air dryers with damp or moist hands will likely reach next for a public restroom doorknob. That is a prescription for the transmission of microbes from one person to another.

The hand-drying story gets more interesting, as different drying methods affect hand contamination—the presence of live bacteria on hands. Warm-air dryers and jet-air dryers were compared with two paper towel types with regard to changes in numbers of bacterial colony forming units (CFUs) on fingertips and palms after washing and drying. In this experiment all volunteers' hands were washed in the same manner and the presence of bacteria tested with multiple methods of bacterial culture. Growing bacteria on a variety of nutrient agar plates reveals the presence of different strains of microbes. When hands were washed and then dried with paper towels, the bacterial count was reduced under all conditions, ranging from a decline of 32.8 percent to a drop of 91.5 percent. (The mean reduction was 76 percent on finger pads and 77 percent on palms.) When hands were washed, then dried with warm-air dryers, the bacterial counts rose in all cases, from +114 percent (a 100 percent increase means that the number of colonies has doubled) to an increase of more than 478 percent (almost five times the prewash count), with mean increases of 194 percent and 254 percent on palms. The implication is, if you wash your hands with soap and water, and then dry with a warm-air dryer, you may end up with hands that are significantly more contaminated. The results of drying hands using the jet dryer were better than the warm-air dryer, but still not as good as paper towels; the jet-air dryer showed an average increase in bacterial colonies of 42 percent on finger pads and 15 percent on palms. In a few cases the jet dryer did decrease bacterial counts, decreasing colony-forming units by 8.4 percent and 11.3 percent in two trials.[92] The jet dryer company markets its product by claiming that it reduces contamination better. In this statement it is likely that they are comparing the jet dryer to other electronic dryers, rather than paper towels.

In the next experiment the researchers asked if paper towels, warm-air dryers, and jet dryers can spread microbes. After all, both electronic methods involve blowing air on wet hands. In the study, they deliberately contaminated volunteers' hands with living yeast cultures; these are yeasts that are typically used for cooking and fermenting beer, so they are innocuous and not disease causing. They were used in order to simulate other microbes that might be found on the hands or in the environment. They randomly assigned the individuals to use four hand-drying approaches: two types of paper towels, a warm-air dryer, or a jet-air dryer, and they collected microbes on culture dishes at various distances from the paper towel dispenser and the dryers. With paper towel drying methods, very few yeast colonies were detected on plates directly under the dispenser. About tenfold higher amounts (thirty-four colonies) were found under the warm-air dryer, and forty-seven colonies were directly under the jet-air dryer. A quarter-meter (about ten inches) away, the colony counts dropped to almost nil for paper towels and for the warm-air dryer, but the jet-air dryer spread more microbes, with seventy-six colonies appearing at that distance from the jet-air dryer. Significant numbers of yeast colonies were collected as far away as two meters from the jet-air dryer unit (over six feet away). The spread of microbes from the jet-air dryer was statistically higher than paper towels for all distances tested. Differences between the warm-air dryer and paper towels were significant in the closest culture dishes. Warm-air versus jet-air dryers differed significantly except at zero meters. The conclusion from this experiment is that warm-air and jet-air dryers can broadcast and spray, or drop germs from drying hands. Warm-air dryers spread mainly in the immediate vicinity, while jet-air dryers, which have powerful fans that blast air as fast as four hundred miles per hour, can spray microbes up to six feet from the unit. They produce and propel aerosols that can suspend microbes in the air which could not only contaminate surfaces, but also be inhaled by people in the washroom.[93]

The final experiment was to analyze microbial contamination on the devices themselves. They tested public restroom jet-air dryers by swabbing the surfaces and growing those contaminants on nutrient agar in the lab. *Staphylococcus aureus*, *E. coli*, and *Pseudomonas aeruginosa* were found on the public washroom jet-air dryers. All of those microbes are potential pathogens; those and other germs from infected people could potentially spread by the powerful jet-air fan blasting air through its narrow slot onto the hands of unsuspecting users and into the restroom environment.[94]

Since that study was not formally peer-reviewed for a journal, I looked at a number of other research reports on the topic of hand drying. A study that was published in a mainstream peer-reviewed journal compared the spread of bacteria from paper towels to an air-blade (aka jet-air) dryer. The results confirmed the earlier study, namely, compared to paper towels, 170,000 more colony-forming units of bacteria were spread on floor surfaces after the use of the air-blade dryer. If used by people whose hands still have germs, there is a good chance the air blade will spread microbes to the washroom environment. "Because the hands are never free of micro-organisms after washing, there is the potential that the choice of drying method will affect the amount of microbial contamination from the wet hands to the surrounding environment during the drying process," noted the authors.[95] Observe that in this article, as in the last study, there existed a potential conflict of interest since the research was supported by SCA Hygiene Products, Göteborg, Sweden, which produces consumer tissue, paper towels, napkins, and toilet paper.[96]

As we have seen, meta-analysis, which compares studies done by different research groups, can help us to better understand complex relationships in scientific studies. Review articles can achieve similar goals, as they also scrutinize the work of a number of researchers in the field. One useful review article compared the data from twelve full research studies on hand drying, comparing paper towels, cloth towels, warm-air dryers, and jet-air dryers.[97] They noted contradictory outcomes; for instance, while some researchers found air dryers to be inferior, others concluded that they are safe and effective. There is a disparity in results from different studies because of varied methodology and different approaches to the issue. However, the authors of this review were able to wade through the various studies and come to some conclusions and consensus based on analysis of all twelve studies. They noted that paper towels may be more effective in reducing bacterial count because drying hands with paper towels relies on friction, and friction can dislodge more bacteria. When used paper towels are tested, researchers find evidence of many bacteria that transferred from the wet hands to the paper. Warm-air and jet-air dryers do not have the advantage of friction—there is no contact with the skin, so they cannot rub germs off the hands. Their second conclusion after analysis of the twelve studies was that air circulation moves microbes around a room, and the fans found in warm-air and jet-air dryers do just that. They can and do disperse infective aerosols. Finally, these electronic devices are easy to contaminate as they are being touched all the time by a succession of wet hands, and the germs harbored in each unit can be spread by the blowing action.[98]

After looking into twelve studies, they conclude that "hot air dryers are generally not recommended for use in health care settings because such dryers are relatively slow and noisy and their hygiene performance is questionable." Neither do the authors like cloth roller towels as "they can become common use towels at the end of the roll." Paper towels are preferred as their use does not generate great air currents. "On the basis of our review, drying hands thoroughly with single-use disposable paper towels is the preferred method of hand drying in terms of hand hygiene."[99] That raises the question of what type of paper towels are best. Recycled paper may be preferred as it has less of a negative impact on the environment. A final recommendation by the authors has to do with the disposal of used paper towels, since the disposal bins can be sources of contamination and could spread microbes. Regular cleaning of washrooms, including the proper disposal of used paper products is of the essence in maintaining control of hygiene when paper products are used.[100]

Once again, let the reader beware, as it is important to note that the authors of the study reported a "Potential Competing Interest." (A number of professional journals insist on this type of disclosure now.) One of the authors, Susan Stack, worked as a consultant for Kimberly-Clark in Sydney, Australia, and Kimberly-Clark is one of the world leaders in the manufacture of, you guessed it, paper towels.

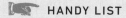 **HANDY LIST**

*The Most Important Times to Wash Your Hands
with Soap and Water*

ESPECIALLY FOR KIDS

1   After using the bathroom
2   After playing with a pet
3   After walking Fido and pooper-scooper duty
4   After playing in the playground
5   After traveling on a bus or subway (public transport)
6   After school
7   After contact sports activities
8   After sneezing or blowing your nose
9   Before touching your eyes
10 After playing in the garden
11 Right before eating

FOR TEENS/ADULTS — ALL OF THE ABOVE, PLUS

1   Before putting in contact lenses
2   Before applying makeup
3   Before using a tampon
4   After gardening

FOR ADULTS — ALL OF THE ABOVE, PLUS

1   Before and after sexual activities
2   After changing a diaper
3   Before preparing food
4   Before feeding a child (or infirm adult)
5   Before tending to a skin lesion or wound
6   After work
7   After working out in the gym

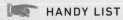 **HANDY LIST**

When to Use Wipes or Alcohol-Based Hand Rubs

1 When no running water is available, that is, on a field trip or outing, any time when you would typically need to wash your hands (see the previous Handy Lists). (When returning to the facilities, hands should be washed with soap and water.)

    At the park

    At the beach

    At a sports event

    When hiking

    When camping

    After shaking hands

    After touching animals

    After using a porta potty

2 During diaper changing, after removing the soiled diaper, the caretaker's hands should be wiped with a wipe before touching the clean diaper or the baby's cleaned skin. (This is recommended with the understanding that washing with soap and water is still preferred, but not practical when handling a wriggling baby on the changing table.)

3 Before touching a wound or skin lesion

4 After encountering body fluids

5 For diabetics, before taking a blood sample or administering insulin

Microbe Hunting
Historic and Biological Roots of Hygiene

For most of human history, people did not wash their hands for the sake of health. It is difficult to imagine that the necessity for hand-washing and other modern hygienic practices, simple acts that we take for granted, was not understood or practiced until the scientific discoveries of the nineteenth century. While there were customs and rituals associated with purity that might have had incidental hygienic effects, the idea of washing hands for health was not part of typical human behavior, and in many parts of the world this is still the case. The early history of hand hygiene mostly involves religious traditions of purity and holiness, rather than cleanliness.

You could argue that people did well enough without practicing basic hygiene. You could argue that, but you would be wrong, because people contracted awful diseases, diseases that were disfiguring, disabling, and deadly. And they did die: the weak and the strong, men, women, and children, young and old, from preventable diseases.

How did humankind learn about microbes and how to stay healthy? It was a very long process, with many skeptics, disbelievers, and those who supported the status quo fighting to stay ignorant. Scientific discoveries made mainly in the last two hundred years were driven by a quest to understand the natural world and the desire to reveal the scientific basis for disease. Now that we have solid empirical evidence for how infectious diseases spread, we can apply that knowledge and improve community and individual health care, and day-to-day health. But the road that led to this knowledge was far from smooth. The pioneers of hygiene had to fight against convention, and some were marginalized, ridiculed, ignored, and even fired from their jobs. Traditional notions were hard to transform; science and scientists were not easily accepted, and human behavior was difficult to change.

To understand our modern attitudes toward hand hygiene, we begin by discussing the roots and origins of hand-hygiene practices found in ancient texts, religions, and rituals. The ancient traditions influenced everyday behavior and human health, in both positive and negative ways. Next we trace hygiene through human history, including the triumphs and failures with regard to hygienic practices. The failures led to disease and death on a massive scale. The triumphs and achievements, spearheaded by courageous scientists, led to progress in managing and defeating infectious disease. Finally, we discuss the biological roots of hygiene, the benign and deadly microbes in our world and how they interact with us.

Religious Roots and Practices

JUDEO-CHRISTIAN ROOTS OF HAND HYGIENE

When my daughter was in nursery school, I had the opportunity to visit the class and observe daily activities. The children came in from the playground, lined up, and were instructed to "wash" their hands by plunging them into a basin of water. One after another, the twenty pairs of hands were submerged in the same basin of water. I cringed when I thought of all the shared dirt and germs in that basin of water and how that approach to washing was not hygienic. I was disappointed by this ignorant approach to hand hygiene; after all, this was a Jewish nursery school class, and handwashing is one of the first religious rituals Jewish children are taught in observant Jewish homes. The approach in that classroom to handwashing did not conform to the practices of modern hygiene, nor did it conform to the practices of Jewish ritual handwashing. Jewish ritual handwashing is never done by immersing the hands in a basin of standing water. It involves pouring clean water from a cup, over the hands, alternating from one hand to the other.

The Biblical origins of handwashing can be found in the Old Testament, dating back 3,400 years. In Exodus (30:17–21) God commanded Moses to make a copper laver, or washbasin, for the priests, Aaron and his sons. "When they go into the tabernacle of the congregation, they shall wash with water, that they die not . . . so shall they wash their hands and their feet, that they die not; and it shall be a statute forever to them, even to him and to his seed throughout their generations." The Biblical text is glaringly clear—wash your hands, or you will die. Handwashing is also described in Deuteronomy (21: 6–7) as part of a ritual carried out by elders of the nearest city in the case when a murder victim is discovered in a field. "And all the elders of that city . . . shall wash their hands . . . and say, 'Our hands have not shed this blood.'" In this case handwashing is a symbolic ritual, declaring the innocence of the town's leaders, who failed to find the perpetrator. These examples emphasize ritual purification as the primary goal of biblical handwashing, but the side benefits of hygiene should not be discounted.

After the destruction of the second Holy Temple in Jerusalem in 70 C.E., rabbinic leaders in the Judaic community adapted some Temple practices to rituals in everyday life. For instance, Temple sacrifices were replaced by synagogue prayer services. In addition, the dinner table in the home was considered analogous to the Temple altar, hence the sages commanded that Jews wash their hands before breaking bread, as the priests washed before offering sacrifices. Since handwashing was part of Temple worship, it became of tremendous importance in many post-Temple rituals. The Talmud, or oral law, a vast compendium of rabbinic commentary on the scripture, has more than three hundred references to handwashing, including descriptions of how to do it, the source of water to use, and when it is needed.

In Talmud Berachot, the notion of washing after defecation was introduced. "R. Yohanan also said: 'If one desires to accept upon himself the yoke of the kingdom of heaven in the most complete manner, he should turn aside, then wash his hands, then put on tefillin [phylacteries], then recite the Shema and say the morning prayers.'"[1] "Turn aside" is a euphemism for defecation, and the best religious practices demanded handwashing after defecation. The practice of washing the hands took on such significance that it was reported that the great sage Rabbi Akiva, when confined to a Roman prison, declared that he would rather die than eat without first washing his hands.[2]

To be sure, not all ancient Israelite practices were health promoting. Clues to the hygienic behavior of an ancient sect are documented in the Dead Sea Scrolls, which revealed the location of the group's latrine. The sect, called the Essenes, lived an ascetic life at Qumran near the Dead Sea in Israel. Because their religious zealotry demanded extreme purity, when they defecated they buried their waste at a site far removed from their living quarters. Archeologists studied the site, whose sandy soil differed from surrounding areas, and discovered that it harbored remnants of intestinal parasites, such as tapeworms, roundworms, and pinworms. When feces are buried in earth, contaminating parasites can survive in the soil for many months, thus infecting and reinfecting members of the sect as they used the latrine. (It is interesting to note that modern Bedouin residents of the region leave their waste out in the open, where the sunlight and heat can disinfect and destroy intestinal parasites and other microbes.) To further amplify the problem, after defecating, the sect members would immerse themselves from head to toe in ritual baths—standing pools of water nearby—before returning to camp. Standing water is an excellent breeding ground for parasites and all sorts of horrible diseases. Analysis of human remains excavated from the Qumran cemetery suggested that the population was, indeed, rife with disease. Based on analysis of the bones, it appears that few of the Essene residents survived to the age of forty, whereas other peoples of that era, living not far from there in Jericho, had longer life expectancies, with a significant number of adult males living beyond the age of forty.[3] Of course, their life expectancy also could have been affected by a number of factors, such as their asceticism, celibacy, desert lifestyle, or diet.

The Essenes lived in ancient Judaea from the second century B.C.E. through the first century C.E., the period of time when Jesus of Nazareth lived. It goes without saying that Jesus and his disciples had an historic impact on culture, traditions, and observances, starting in ancient Judaea and spreading worldwide. But what is less appreciated is that handwashing, among other practices, became a controversial political and religious issue in the time of Jesus. According to the Gospel of Mark, the Pharisees and scribes left Jerusalem and met up with Jesus and his disciples, "And when they saw some of his disciples eat bread with defiled, that is to say, with unwashen, hands, they found fault" (Mark 7:2).

Commentators explain that Jesus "set aside ceremonial law," including handwashing before meals. One Christian commentator, Matthew Henry, explains Jesus's message of "clean hands and pure heart" as being symbolic of how to worship God and relate to fellow men, not as a literal obligation to wash hands.[4]

John Gill's commentary discusses how the laws of the Scribes, considered by Jewish sources as the Oral Tradition, were strictly followed by Jews in the days of Jesus. Gill quotes from the Talmud to illustrate the severity of the laws, "R. Jose says, 'whoever eats bread without washing of hands, is as if he lay with a whore': and, says R. Eleazer, 'whoever despiseth washing of hands, shall be rooted out of the world.'"[5] The break of Christianity with rabbinic traditions, including the disciples eating with unwashed hands, was emblematic of the greater breach of Christianity with the Jewish leadership. Gill explains that this was one way "they distinguished a Jew from a Gentile; if he washed his hands, and blessed, he was known to be an Israelite, but if not, a Gentile."[6] So how important was handwashing back in those days? It was a symbolic and ritual act so significant that the change in attitude and action with regard to handwashing represented the movement toward a new world religion. It is important to note that the link between handwashing and health was not scientifically established until the nineteenth century; it was rabbinic ritual that was being rejected, not hygiene.

Water in Christian Religious Ritual

In Christianity today, while rites and rituals vary from denomination to denomination, to most adherents baptism is the major Christian sacrament that involves purification with water. It commemorates the baptism of Jesus by John the Baptist in the Jordan River and represents the washing away of sins. For Eastern Orthodox Christians water and olive oil are both important in church rituals, and their baptism ceremony involves the total immersion of the infant (or adult) in water, followed by anointing with oil. Passages that are recited reflect the ritual purification role of the water. "But do You, O Master of All, declare this water to be water of redemption, water of sanctification, a cleansing of flesh and spirit, a loosing of bonds, a forgiveness of sins, an illumination of soul, a laver of regeneration, a renewal of the spirit, a gift of sonship, a garment of incorruption, a fountain of life. For You have said, O Lord: 'Wash, and be clean; put away evil from your souls.'"[7] In Catholicism there are varied approaches to baptism, or christening, that is, the symbolic washing away of sin: full or partial immersion in water, or affusion, which is pouring of water on the forehead, followed by anointing with oil. Baptists, Jehovah's Witnesses, Latter Day

Saints, and the Church of Christ all practice baptism by complete immersion in baptismal fonts, swimming pools, bathtubs, creeks, or rivers.

Water plays a role in other Christian rituals as well. People of the Greek Orthodox faith celebrate the Feast of the Theophany on January 6 (or according to the Julian calendar still used by some Orthodox churches, on January 19), commemorating the baptism of Jesus with the "Great Blessing of Water." The church and congregation are blessed with holy water, and in the days following, the priest visits the homes of the parishioners to bless the families and their homes with holy water.

In the early days of Christianity, two to three centuries after Christ, the *lavabo* (Latin for "I wash myself"), a ritual handwashing vessel and bowl, was introduced as part of church service. Eastern Christians still maintain the lavabo outside of the refectory. In Roman Catholic churches, after the clergy don ceremonial vestments (clerical clothing) the priest washes his hands in the lavabo and says prayers.

In the Communion ceremony, the priest's hands are washed by acolytes or altar boys. In many churches the sprinkling of holy water on hands takes place before the consecration of bread and wine, and in Catholicism, hands are washed after handling Holy Oil.[8] In some Roman Catholic churches, there are lavers that may be used by congregants to ritually cleanse themselves. Fingers are dipped into the holy water, and the sign of the cross is made.

If you travel around the Middle East wearing sandals, you may appreciate why foot washing was important to ancient peoples living in that part of the world, as there is a lot of dust and sand, and feet get filthy. Foot washing was part and parcel of ancient hospitality, and a gracious host would welcome guests by providing water to wash their feet, as well as food and drink. In modern religious practice, once a year many Christians perform ritual washing of the feet on Maundy (Holy) Thursday, recalling the Last Supper when Jesus washed the feet of his twelve apostles. Every year the Pope performs the ritual washing of the feet as a sign of his humility, choosing the most simple and humble of people to perform it on. Many Christian denominations, including Eastern Orthodox, Catholics, and Protestants, carry out different variations of the washing of the feet. While not directly relevant to hand hygiene, this practice does give us insight into ancient attitudes about hygiene and the importance of water.

Jewish Ritual Handwashing

Ritual handwashing, *netilat yadayim*, has retained significance in modern Jewish observance. Observant Jews wash before eating any bread, and make the blessing, "Blessed art Thou, Lord our God, King of the universe, who has sanctified us with His commandments, and commanded us to wash hands." A special cup with two handles is typically used. The cup is filled with water, and the water is poured two or three times over each hand. In the spirit of enhancing Jewish practice, it is now possible to purchase beautifully crafted and artistically decorated washing cups, many of which are made in Israel. It is common for a newly engaged Orthodox Jewish couple to receive a washing cup (or two) as a gift for their new home.

Some Jews also practice handwashing after the meal. The so-called "last waters," or *mayim acharonim*, is believed to have originated for health reasons. Before refrigeration was invented, a large amount of salt was used to preserve food. If the fingers had salt residue after eating, touching the eyes could cause eye irritation or even blindness, so rinsing the fingers after eating was implemented. There are special tiny pitchers and bowls used for this après dinner ritual.

Handwashing is also practiced as part of the morning wake-up ritual. Observant Jews will, upon awakening in the morning, rinse their hands with *negel vasser* (literally "nail water"). Judaism teaches that during the night the soul leaves the body and is returned by God every morning. Handwashing is the first act performed in the morning, to purify the person in case he has touched private areas of the body, and to sanctify and prepare the person for service to God.

Ritual handwashing is practiced by many Jews after touching objects that could convey impurity, such as leather shoes or ritually unclean animals, or after visiting a cemetery. Ritual handwashing also may be performed after using the bathroom, cutting one's nails or hair, touching the genitalia, or having a seminal emission. In addition, in the synagogue service, before the *kohanim* (priests, that is, Jews who trace their lineage to Aaron the biblical high priest) bless the congregation, they remove their shoes and then have their hands ritually washed by Levites (individuals in the congregation who are descendants of the tribe of Levi).

Today we would hope that everyone knows enough about hygiene to wash their hands before eating. However, it is not always convenient to do so, and I have observed many people who fail to do any washing immediately before "breaking bread." But when modern observant Jews eat, they are still required to ritually wash their hands before eating bread; and as we have seen, the act of ritual washing with plain water can reduce bacteria and have positive effects on health. Ritual handwashing raises awareness of hand hygiene in general, and it also may influence people to more scrupulously wash with soap and water before a meal. Thus, the Biblical injunction to "wash with water that they die not" and rabbinic interpretations of the ancient traditions on handwashing contribute to the spiritual as well as physical health of individuals in the Jewish community. I suspect that my own father, a rabbi who developed meticulous hygiene practices, was strongly influenced by his Jewish upbringing, his scholarship and learning of scripture and Talmud, and their emphasis on hand hygiene.

WASHING RITUALS IN ISLAM

Purification and washing is a major tenet of Islam, historically the third major monotheistic world religion to emerge. The Islamic prophet Mohammed led his followers in the seventh century to embrace the worship of Allah, following their holy book, the Qur'an. "Personal cleanliness is paramount to worship in Islam."[9] Indeed, during the Dark Ages in Europe, the Islamic world cultivated individuals of scientific insight and medical acuity. The Islamic physician and chemist Muhammad ibn Zakariyā Rāzī, also known as Rhazes, studied infectious diseases and wrote a highly respected treatise on smallpox and measles, demonstrating his use of scientific observation and concluding that those two diseases are distinct and different. Born in Persia in 865, Rāzī later moved to Baghdad and became a prominent physician and director of one of the first hospitals established in the Islamic world. He was a thousand years ahead of his time, espousing egalitarian and antiauthoritarian principles, and supporting freedom of inquiry, and he carried out these principles by offering medical treatment to princes and paupers alike. This approach did not make him popular among the Islamic religious leaders, whose authority was generally unquestioned. Rāzī was a prolific writer who wrote scholarly books on a wide range of topics in astronomy, alchemy, medicine, philosophy, and mathematics; those works served as guides for medical practice, science, and philosophical thought for hundreds of years.[10]

Mohammed ibn Hasan ibn Ali Abu Ja'far al-Tusi, a Shi'ite jurist on Islamic law who lived from 995–1066 C.E., wrote a comprehensive guide to Islamic Law, which opens with "The Book of Physical Cleanliness (*taharah*) and Ablution."[11] One section, devoted to "Water as a Cleaning Agent and the Rulings Concerning It," demonstrates a sophisticated understanding of hygiene with regard to water safety. It defines two types of water: unadulterated water (*mutlaq*), which is clean and cleanses, and adulterated water (*mudaf*), which is clean but cannot cleanse. Adulterated water includes water that is extracted from fruits or vegetables or is left over from cooking. Unadulterated water can be either running water or stagnant water. All types of running water are considered pure unless they "change colour, taste or smell due to mixing with something impure (*najis*), for example, blood." Pure running water is the best to use for cleansing and ritual purification. Stagnant water is found in pits, puddles, pools, ponds, containers, and wells. If the volume of the stagnant water is small, it can be easily adulterated. If it is a large volume, more than a Kurr (376 liters), then it is pure "unless an impure substance . . . changes its colour, taste or smell."[12]

The book goes on in great detail to give examples of situations that will render water impure. For instance, "If a dog drinks out of a vessel the water becomes ritually impure and must be thrown away. In this case the vessel or container must be washed and rinsed three times, the first time of which should be with soil." In addition, the author instructs, "If an alcoholic substance or semen or menstrual blood drips or is dropped in [a well] or if an animal falls and dies in it, the well must be drained completely. If it is too difficult to do this then four men in turn must keep emptying it for a full day. If a human being dies in a well then seventy average sized buckets of water must be drawn from the well."[13]

We now know scientifically how bodily fluids and dead bodies can transmit disease, and apparently in that society contamination from bodily fluids and dead bodies also was understood to be a risk. In addition, the author cautions, "It is recommended to leave a space of five *dhar's* between a well whose water is used for drinking, and between a cesspool used for sewage purposes. This is in areas where the land is hard and in the case where the well is above (in terms of degrees) the cesspool, otherwise the space between them must be seven *dhar's* in circumference round the well."[14] A *dhar* is 41 inches (104 cm), so the recommended spacing is a minimum of 17 to 24 feet between the well and the cesspool. While they were unaware of microbes a thousand years ago when this was written, these recommendations and policies no doubt helped to keep the community healthy.

In Islam, proscriptions on impurity require purification rites for body and clothes, called *taharah*. (The word *taharah* also means purity in Hebrew, and refers to Jewish ritual purification.) There are two main types of purification: *Ghusl*, or full-body washing, and *Wudu*, or partial ablution, which is performed before *salat*, prayer, five times a day. Pure water from a river, sea, or pond, melting snow or ice, a well or a spring can be used for Wudu or Ghusl. Sunni and Shia Muslims differ in some protocols, but Wudu generally includes the washing of the hands and arms including the elbows, the face, part of the head, and the feet including the ankles. Nostrils and mouth also may be washed, and prayers are chanted during the washing. If no water is available, it is possible to perform Wudu by *Tayammum*, a "dry ablution," which involves rubbing dust or soil over the skin. The purification may be invalidated after defecation, urination, emission of flatulence or semen, or sexual contact, and the *taharah* must be performed again before prayer and before handling and reading the holy book of the Qur'an.[15]

To fulfill the need for ritual washing, mosques have washing facilities, including a foot wash. At larger mosques, such as the Dome of the Rock in Jerusalem, there are hand and foot wash facilities with numerous faucets to serve large numbers of worshippers. The University of Michigan–Dearborn, where more than 10 percent of the student body is Muslim, installed foot-washing stations in some bathrooms on campus to accommodate students who needed those facilities for religious ritual washing. The university presented the facilities as a health and safety measure, and not a violation of the separation of church and state, since washing feet in a regular sink can be awkward and hazardous.[16]

BAHA'I ABLUTIONS

A major principle of the Baha'i religion is purity, hence washing of hands and face is an important ritual that precedes the obligatory prayers several times each day. This religion had its roots in Shi'a Islam in 1844, but now declares itself to be an independent world religion.

While washing hands, people of the Baha'i faith recite, "Whoso wisheth to pray, let him wash his hands." While washing the face, they recite, "I have turned my face unto Thee, O my Lord." The water that is used must be pure, and there are prescriptions for how to determine if it is suitable to use. For instance, "small quantities of water, such as one cupful, or even two or three, must be considered used after a single washing of the face and hands. But a kurr or more of water remaineth unchanged after one or two washings of the face, and there is no objection to its use unless it is altered in one of the three ways." If the color, taste, or smell of the water has changed, it is no longer suitable for ritual washing.[17]

On a Baha'i prayer website, Living Waters, they explain the customs concerning washing and prayer throughout the day. Adherents have written in to the website to ask practical as well as spiritual questions. One person asks what is the best place to perform the ablutions—kitchen or bathroom? The response is that people use either one. Blogger Paul Mantle explains: "I perform mine in the bathroom. I speculate that in the future —though probably not in my lifetime—many homes even in our culture will be designed to better accommodate devotional ablutions; even now some homes have a separate washroom, or an alcove for the sink . . . An appealing option for ablutions might be the use of a pitcher and washbowl on a chest of drawers, nightstand, or low dresser in one's bedroom."[18]

WASHING RITUALS IN OTHER RELIGIONS AND CULTURES

A Sanskrit document from 2000 B.C.E. prescribed the boiling of water in order to purify it.[19] This greatly preceded the understanding of the germ theory, which did not emerge for almost four more millennia. Indian physicians made many other contributions of note. Sushruta, who is thought to have lived between 1200 and 600 B.C.E, studied and documented hundreds of diseases, noting with great foresight the relationship between malaria and mosquitoes.[20] Charaka, who lived in Northern India sometime between 500 B.C.E. to 200 C.E., proposed the concept of inheritance (genetics) through sperm and eggs. He emphasized health and hygiene, encouraging cleanliness to stay healthy, and he believed that diseases were not supernatural, but were due to natural causes.[21]

Hinduism today subscribes to rituals and rites of purification. In India, bathing in the Holy Ganges is a major act of faith, performed before festivals or after there is a death in the community. The Achamana ritual involves touching and sipping pure holy water while reciting mantras. The *kindi* is a water vessel used in Hindi ceremonies, such as the Puja worship. Kindi are typically attractive metal vessels with a long spout; some are kept in the home to wash hands and feet. Some Hindi, who avoid the use of animal products, may reject soap as it may contain animal fat, and instead cleanse hands by rubbing vigorously with mud or ash and rinsing with water. Surprisingly, as we learned in chapter 1, a study done in Bangladesh found that this approach for handwashing is, under some conditions, as effective as soap and water in reducing fecal bacterial contamination.[22] Traditional Hindi principles involve washing before and after meals and after using the toilet.[23]

According to the World Health Organization, "Specific indications regarding hand hygiene are nonexistent in the Buddhist faith."[24] Two symbolic acts in Buddhism involve handwashing, but they are not related to personal hygiene. Buddhists will pour water over the hands of a deceased person before cremation. In addition, it is customary while celebrating the New Year for a younger person to pour water "over the hands of elders to wish them good health and a long life."[25]

The *misogi* of the Japanese Shinto religion is a form of ritual purification that involves immersion in running water. In Japan people travel to lakes, streams, rivers, and waterfalls, where they pray for spiritual purification by immersion or by drinking the water. They wear white ceremonial garb, including headbands. Shintoism, which originated more than two thousand years ago, far from the three monotheistic religions in the Middle East and Europe, also developed water rituals to wash away sins and misfortunes.[26] Suijin, a Shinto *kami*, or water deity, is believed to be found near waterways, springs, lakes, ponds, and wells.[27] Clearly "cleanliness is next to godliness" is a common principle of humankind.

RITUAL WASHING AND HEALTH

Rituals from cultural and religious practices may have contributed in many ways to health. As we have seen, modern medical research has clearly demonstrated the benefits of washing hands after using the bathroom and before eating. Many studies have shown that washing hands with soap and water improves health by reducing the incidence of infectious diseases. For instance, scientists at the University of Michigan School of Public Health conducted an analysis of thirty studies on hand hygiene. The data showed that improvements in hand hygiene reduced the incidence of gastrointestinal illness by 31 percent and respiratory illness by 21 percent.[28] Of course, the critical question is whether washing with plain water, as is done in many types of ritual washing, reduces contamination with microorganisms. In particular, is ritual handwashing effective in reducing infection? There are places on the globe where soap is a luxury, so this question is of more than academic interest, and has serious health-related implications for many people.

A Bangladeshi study cited in chapter 1 found that compared with households where no handwashing took place, households in which mothers washed only one hand or both hands with plain water before food preparation had reduced rates of diarrhea in their children.[29] Because of the cost and inconvenience of using soap in these rural areas, the authors conclude: "The finding from this study . . . suggest[s] that promoting handwashing exclusively with soap may be unwarranted. Handwashing with water alone might be seen as a step on the handwashing ladder; handwashing with water is good; handwashing with soap is better."[30]

A British study also cited in chapter 1 confirmed that water alone can reduce hand contamination. Volunteers were instructed to touch public surfaces in buses, the Underground, and the British Museum, and then wash with soap and water, water alone, or not at all. Bacteria of fecal origin was found on 44 percent of unwashed hands, on 8 percent of hands washed with soap and water, and on 23 percent of hands washed with water alone. This shows that our modern conventional approach to hygiene, washing with soap and water, is highly effective (although not perfect), and water alone, although not as effective as soap and water, can significantly reduce contamination, from 44 percent to 23 percent of samples.[31]

The ancient people using ritual handwashing were on to something. Rinsing hands with water alone reduces bacteria on hands, which in turn may have reduced rates of infection and helped to keep the community healthy. Ritual handwashing that calls for flowing water—water poured over the hands, or from a flowing source, rather than immersion of hands into stagnant water, is likely to even further reduce the risk of infection and transmission of disease.

Epidemics
Hygiene Failures in History

Despite religions and faiths valiantly attempting to keep communities spiritually and physically healthy through a variety of water-based ablutions, disease and untimely death punctuated human history in dramatic fashion. The word *hygiene* is derived from Hygieia, who was the Greek goddess of health and cleanliness. She was the daughter of Asclepius, the god of medicine. Ancient Greek society worshipped gods of health and medicine, and emphasized a regimen of health and personal hygiene. Between 600 and 400 B.C.E., Greek commerce thrived, Athens grew, and they invested in infrastructure to provide public water supplies through cisterns and conduits, as well as public fountains and bathhouses.[32] But even these noble endeavors could not prevent calamity in the form of disease.

The word *epidemic*, which refers to the outbreak of infectious disease, is from the Greek *epi*, or upon, and *demos*, people. An epidemic involves the rapid spreading of a communicable disease through a human population. Despite the emphasis on health and hygiene, and the "protection" of their gods of medicine and cleanliness, ancient Greece suffered calamitous losses when the Plague of Athens tore through that ancient city during the Peloponnesian War in 430 B.C.E. The historian Thucydides described mass death in the crowded living conditions of Athens, how caregivers contracted the disease at very high rates, and how societal norms broke down in the face of massive fatalities in the community. It is estimated that the disease killed as many as two-thirds of the population. There have been speculations about the cause of the epidemic, including viral hemorrhagic fever, such as Ebola; other viruses such as smallpox or measles; or bacterial diseases such as anthrax, typhus, and typhoid fever.

One clue to solving the mystery of what caused the epidemic came from a study of teeth, which can retain cellular material preserved in the pulp cavity for thousands of years. Teeth recovered from an ancient burial pit of that era showed evidence of infection with *Salmonella enterica* subtype *typhi*, the disease-causing organism of typhoid fever.[33] While still under dispute, it is the only physical evidence available; other proposals were based on Thucydides's descriptions of the epidemic conditions and comparisons with other epidemics. Although also uncertain, it is presumed that typhoid fever, caused by food and water contaminated with *Salmonella enterica* subtype *typhi*, was also a cause of death for Alexander the Great, who died a century later at the age of thirty-three, after contracting a fever that lasted eleven days.[34]

Hundreds of years later in the first millennium C.E., plagues decimated populations throughout Europe, Western Asia, and North Africa. The term *decimate* literally means to reduce by a factor of ten; and although exact death tolls are not available, the dramatic loss of human life warrants the use of the hyperbole "decimate." The Romans, who like the Greeks worshipped health and hygiene and built even more advanced aqueducts, sewers for waste management, and public baths, also faced catastrophe when the Antonine Plague struck. It spread through the vast Roman Empire from the years 165 to 180, killing between a third and half of the population. The most likely candidates for causative agents of that epidemic were the smallpox virus or the Rickettsia bacteria that causes typhus.[35]

The Greeks and Romans dedicated tremendous resources to hygiene through bathing; however, the public bath facilities were designed "for reasons of pleasure, politics and propaganda, not disease prevention." Although they worshipped cleanliness, the impact of public baths on health may have been insignificant or marginal. The facilities were difficult to keep clean, and they did not separate sick people from healthy people, so public baths may have contributed to spreading infectious disease.[36]

The next major plague, the Plague of Justinian (541–542) wiped out 25 percent or more of the population of Europe. Bubonic plague, which is transmitted from infected rodents to people via infected fleas, is suspected to have caused that epidemic.[37] The Roman Empire soon slid into obscurity, and "as the Roman Empire broke up, much of the understanding of the need for effective public sanitation was lost. The ruling principle of early Christian Europe was in many ways obedience to authority . . . The hierarchy of the Church also stressed curing the ills of the soul rather than those of the body."[38] Europe entered the Dark Ages, where scientific progress was impeded by politics, religion, and demographics, and science took a back seat to religious authoritarian rule. Many beautiful structures, Roman aqueducts and amphitheaters, from Aegyptus and Judea to Britannia, fell into disrepair as the empire disintegrated.

During the second millennium C.E., from 1346–1353, another major cataclysm struck humanity. The "Black Death," which was attributed to bubonic plague, raged through the population "eventually spreading through the whole of Europe, Asia and North Africa. The disease hit almost every city, town, village and hamlet, wiping out nearly half the inhabitants, and causing the most dramatic fall in population ever recorded."[39]

"Crowds, filth and poverty"[40] were major agents in these historic catastrophes, in which cities teeming with people had insufficient infrastructure to provide clean water or manage waste. The aqueducts and baths of the Greeks and Romans failed to keep the population safe. And the squalor of Europe led to unimaginable suffering and death. While we know that ancient peoples had high mortality rates attributable to disease, these extreme examples highlight the importance of all we have learned about germs and hygiene, mostly from the scientists of the past two hundred years, the so-called "Microbe Hunters."

Microbe Hunters
A New Hope

Europe emerged from dark times into the Renaissance. In the fifteenth and sixteenth centuries, science and medicine were roused and inspired, with brave men exploring the globe and discovering "new" lands and creative scientists exploring nature and discovering new microscopic life. (Ruthless governments and explorers also exploited the newly discovered lands and their inhabitants.) In 1546 Girolamo Fracastoro of Italy proposed that *seminaria*, or invisible seeds, cause disease, formulating for the first time the germ theory of disease. He explained in his writings "On Contagion and Contagious Diseases" that each disease is caused by a unique type of seed, which can grow quickly and can move from person to person through the air, or can be acquired by direct contact with infected materials that he called *fomes*.[41] As we will discuss in chapter 4, *fomites*, a word derived from Fracastoro's *fomes*, are contaminated surfaces that harbor microbes and serve as a vector to transmit disease. Although it took another three hundred years before Pasteur and Koch provided the scientific data that confirmed Fracastoro's notion, the seeds of his ideas and insight inspired other microbe hunters and advanced the understanding of biology and medicine.

In his classic book *Microbe Hunters*, Paul de Kruif weaves the tales of the great scientists from the seventeenth through the early twentieth centuries, who discovered the microbial basis for disease. They were pioneers, people of vision, and mavericks who challenged the superstitions of their day, carefully examining the natural world and developing empirical approaches to study and test their hypotheses. World travel and the development of routes to and from new corners of the world sadly also led to the emergence of new epidemics. The venereal disease syphilis and other afflictions spread like wildfire from brothel to bedroom, to rich and poor, peasant and royalty. The world needed "these microbe hunters and death fighters," who were "bold and persistent and curious explorers." They were the innovators, who spent lonely days and nights with "tireless peerings into this new fantastic world."[42]

First published in 1926, *Microbe Hunters* was reprinted dozens of times. My little paperback edition, handed down to me by my older brother, is the thirtieth paperback printing, dated 1964. The yellowed pages are cracking and in danger of disintegrating, but still hold the tales of the curious and brave scientists who made wondrous discoveries.

How did these men become microbe hunters? Antony van Leeuwenhoek (1632–1723) was a Dutchman from Delft, from a family of basket makers and brewers. He left school at the age of sixteen; after training as an apprentice in a dry goods store, he opened his own store, and later on became a janitor at the city hall. In his spare time, he developed a passion for grinding lenses and an obsession for looking through them. So with little formal education, he began his own quest to study the world of the very, very tiny. He mounted hundreds of his perfect lenses in tubes and built the best microscopes of the time. Like a man possessed, he looked at everything he could think of in his new devices: a bee's stinger, louse legs, beaver hairs. His discoveries got even more interesting when he looked at rainwater, plain ordinary rainwater. De Kruif reenacts his version of Leeuwenhoek's breakthrough, relating the exclamations of Leeuwenhoek: "Come here! Hurry! There are little animals in this rain water . . . They swim! They play around! They are a thousand times smaller than any creatures we can see with our eyes alone . . . Look! See what I have discovered!"[43]

Leeuwenhoek's descriptions of the living creatures taken from his own mouth revealed many aspects of the microbial world. He took some material from between his teeth and mixed it with rainwater or with his own spittle. "Then to my great surprise I perceived that the . . . matter contained very many small living Animals, which moved themselves very extravagantly. The biggest sort had the shape of A. Their motion was strong & nimble, and they darted themselves thro the water or spittle, as a Jack or a Pike does thro the water." He observed ovals, circles, and some that "spun like a top." He observed "Animals" taken from between the teeth of several women, an eight-year-old child, and two old men. He noted that drinking brandy, wine, or using tobacco did not kill the "animals," and neither did gargling with wine vinegar. But mixing the creatures directly with wine vinegar did kill them. He correctly noted that "the number of these Animals in the scurf of a mans Teeth, are so many that I believe they exceed the number of Men in a kingdom."[44]

Leeuwenhoek needed to know where the "wretched beasties" came from, so he designed an experiment to catch pure, uncontaminated rainwater, and found no creatures at all growing in the fresh water. But after the water sat outside for several days, it was teeming with microscopic life. "They do not come from the sky," he concluded, rather from impurities blown in and settling in from the environment. He reported his findings to the Royal Society of England: He had discovered microbes in drinking water, in the mouth, in the guts of animals, in oysters, and in many other sources. He demonstrated for the first time how to kill microbes, when he learned that hot coffee killed the beasties in his mouth. Leeuwenhoek worked well into his eighties, continuing to explore and report his findings and making discoveries that were astounding for his time. Even on his deathbed, at age ninety-one, he instructed that his final reports be sent to London, to the Royal Society, to share with the world.[45]

The Italian Lazzaro Spallanzani (1729–1799), born just a few years after Leeuwenhoek's death, was an ordained priest with a scientific mind. He was captivated by Leeuwenhoek's work and convinced that the smallest creatures arose not from thin air, that is, by spontaneous generation, which was the prevailing view of the day, but from other microscopic life. Spallanzani is best remembered for designing an elegant experiment where boiled, sterilized broth is sealed into flasks by melting the glass neck shut. Under those conditions, no living creatures appear. In similar flasks left open, or closed only with corks, the broth is teeming with microscopic "animalcules." Spallanzani concluded that life comes only from preexisting life; it does not originate spontaneously from inanimate matter.

In the course of his experiments, Spallanzani also learned that there are different classes of *animalcula*, some of which are very sensitive to heat ("boiling for a single second prevented their existence") and some that are highly resistant to heat, which were most likely bacteria that form heat-resistant spores. He noted the diversity of microbes from different environments, and even from the same type of culture repeated on different occasions. "The *animalcula* of the same infusion were different, at different times and different places . . . All this well agrees with the vast variety of animalcular eggs, scattered in the air, and falling ever where, without any law . . . The idea, that *animalcula* come from the air, appears to me to be confirmed by undoubted facts."[46]

In addition, he observed and reported on something considered at that time to be impossible, that some kinds of microbes could live without air. We now know of many classes of anaerobes, microbes that derive energy in the absence of oxygen. *Bacteroides fragilis* is one example of anaerobic bacteria that can cause infection in humans. It is associated with appendicitis and other infections that occur in places with access to little oxygen; those types of infections are hard to eradicate.

Finally, according to de Kruif, when Spallanzani read a report on how microbes reproduce, he had to see it for himself. He isolated a single animalcule and observed it in the microscope splitting into two separate creatures, a process we now call binary fission. Thus, he was one of the first to observe and report on bacterial reproduction.[47]

Despite these dramatic discoveries, it still took many decades for the field to have practical application in improving human health. The era of medical hand hygiene arose formally in 1847, in a Vienna hospital, where Professor Ignaz Semmelweis (1818–1865) discovered that doctors who went from performing autopsies directly to maternity wards were spreading deadly disease to pregnant women. In those days it was common practice for doctors to move from ward to ward, lab to clinic, and from dead bodies to live patients, without washing hands, and this practice was calamitous. Mortality rates soared, and one in ten, or even as many as one in four women, died from complications related to childbirth in that hospital. Semmelweis noticed that the two maternity wards in Vienna's General

Hospital, both of which treated comparable numbers of cases, differed dramatically in mortality rates. In the ward where midwives delivered babies there were typically about sixty deaths per year. In the ward where obstetricians and medical students delivered babies the mortality rate was at least ten times higher, with six hundred to eight hundred deaths. One difference between the wards was that doctors and students were required to perform autopsies daily on maternity patients who had died. The doctors would frequently find themselves rushing directly from the morgue to a woman in labor.[48]

Semmelweis's close friend, pathologist Jakob Kolletschka, also performed such autopsies. One day he accidentally cut his finger during a procedure; within days he came down with a raging fever and died. Semmelweis realized that his friend's symptoms matched those of childbed fever (also known as puerperal fever), which was plaguing the maternity wards, and that the punctured finger could have served as the pathway for transmission. In those days doctors did not yet understand how infectious microbes caused disease, but Semmelweis had the insight to suggest a connection between a breach in the skin and transfer of the disease from a cadaver to his friend. Semmelweis noted, "The fact of the matter was that the transmitting source of the cadaver particles was to be found in the hands of the students and attending physicians."[49]

This raging epidemic of childbed fever was hospital propagated. In Semmelweis's lecture on the origin of the disease, he noted that "before the establishment of the general hospital (1784) . . . there was no extensive epidemic of puerperal fever, and the death rate was below 1 percent."[50] Semmelweis instituted a handwashing protocol for doctors that significantly reduced the mortality rate in the maternity ward. He managed to convince the hospital administration to require doctors and students to disinfect hands in a solution of chlorinated lime before they entered the maternity ward. Mortality rates for new mothers dropped from 18.3 percent to 1.2 percent, saving hundreds of lives in the first year of implementation.[51]

Sadly, Semmelweis's insight and success were not welcomed with open arms by other doctors, because his ideas contradicted conventional wisdom and the practices of the day. Years later President Woodrow Wilson wisely noted, "If you want to make enemies, try to change something." Even though Semmelweis had proven that his approach worked to reduce mortality, he and his followers struggled to convince his colleagues and to gain acceptance of even the most rudimentary approaches to hygiene. He was thwarted by resistance and politics, and when his assistantship ended, he was not reappointed at the hospital. He protested, fought, and defended his theory, but the entrenched powers prevailed. Semmelweis returned to a small hospital in his homeland of Hungary, where by implementing the new policies he reduced maternal mortality rates to below 1 percent. But he was still frustrated and angry, bitter and obsessed; and this led to deep depression and mania, commitment to an asylum, and an untimely death at the age of forty-seven.[52]

Louis Pasteur's reputation as a microbe hunter was established by his many published works and extraordinary achievements, and his work has been documented in many books on science history. The brilliance and insight of this man cannot be overstated. He changed our understanding of many areas of biology; in fact, his work led to the development of new fields of study, as well as dramatic progress in the fledgling fields of biology, medicine, infectious disease, health, hygiene, and immunology. His research not only had applications in medicine, but also in commercial areas such as alcoholic brewing and silk production. You could say that his discoveries even laid a foundation for the modern biotechnology industry. Today Pasteur's name appears on every carton of milk and orange juice, as he discovered that heating beverages, a process we call pasteurization, kills microbes that can make us sick. This standard of food preparation keeps us healthy today.

In the early 1800s the link between the microscopic world and disease was yet to be established. Pasteur was the one to reveal the microbial cause of disease. Louis Pasteur (1822–1895) was a young boy when a rabid wolf attacked residents of his French village, and he is said to have been greatly distressed by seeing the suffering and agonizing deaths of the victims. In his early schooling in Paris he discovered chemistry, and his scientific abilities as a young investigator led him to discover features of crystals and the three-dimensional shapes of molecules that laid the groundwork for organic chemistry (the same organic chemistry that every pre-med struggles with). Soon he turned his attention to the biochemistry of alcoholic fermentation, which led to his passion for studying microscopic organisms. In the course of helping a local beet-sugar distiller whose stills were producing acid instead of alcohol, Pasteur observed that in the healthy vats where sugars were converted into the desired alcoholic beverage, there were globular organisms, the yeasts.[53] This confirmed the earlier work of Charles Cagniard-Latour, who first linked living yeast cells to the production of alcohol. Cagniard-Latour had reported on the reproduction of beer yeast, "organized microscopic bodies which are very simple," and had proposed correctly that yeast convert sugar into carbon dioxide and alcohol.[54]

But Pasteur had to solve the brewers' problem. In the vats where a putrid, acidic product was made, he found no yeasts, rather he discovered contaminating "rods," bacteria that spoil the fermentation process. Based on his work, he was able to advise the brewers on how to optimize their alcohol production by nurturing yeast cells and eliminating contaminating bacteria. Pasteur's work improved the brewing industry, which helped the production of world-renowned French wines and even improved the notoriously unremarkable French beer. His meticulous experiments on fermentation also showed that it was yeast cells on the outside of grape skin that achieved fermentation of wine, and those yeast cells could be collected to use in other fermentation processes as well.[55]

Another world-changing contribution by Pasteur was his pioneering discovery and development of aseptic packaging. By boiling milk and other beverages, and then sealing up the bottles, he was able to preserve them for years without spoilage. We use these principles today for preserving foods in sterile aseptic packages, such as cans, sealed jars, and more recently sealed aseptic bags and pouches.

Pasteur had other triumphant accomplishments in microbiology. For instance, when he was asked to rescue the silk industry in the south of France, after six years of painstaking work, he discovered two parasitic diseases that attack silkworms. He then taught the farmers how to avoid propagating the diseases and save the industry.[56]

A century had passed since Spallanzani had disproved spontaneous generation, concluding that microscopic life comes from other microbes. But Spallanzani's original experiment did not convince all of the scientific community, as it was flawed. Perhaps the microbes failed to grow in his sealed flasks because they were deprived of natural air, which, his critics reasoned, was essential for life. One of Pasteur's most famous experiments was a variation on Spallanzani's original experiment that had disproved spontaneous generation a century earlier. Pasteur repeated Spallanzani's experiment with one adjustment: the broth would be incubated in flasks designed to permit access to air. Pasteur drew sketches of his unique vessels—flasks with long, thin necks, curved like the neck of a swan. When broth or milk inside the new vessels were boiled sterile, the liquid could remain uncontaminated for many days, even though the long, curved neck was open to the air. Because of the curved glass neck, airborne microbes could not fall in and contaminate the liquid. The broth in these oddly shaped flasks remained clear and free of microbes, despite being open to the environment. "At this moment," wrote Pasteur, "I have in my laboratory many highly alterable liquids which have remained unchanged for 18 months in open vessels with curved or inclined necks." Indeed, this experiment "proves without doubt that the origin of life, in infusions which have been boiled, arises uniquely from the solid particles which are suspended in the air . . . bodies which cannot be distinguished from true germs of the organisms of infusions." In other words, life does not come out of thin air or from sterile broth; only microscopic life begets life.[57]

The English surgeon, Joseph Lister, was impressed with Pasteur's work and credited it with helping him implement antiseptic practices in hospitals and clinics. Lister himself made great inroads in the control of infections in hospitals with his introduction of carbolic acid as an antiseptic. His 1867 publication "On the Antiseptic Principle in the Practice of Surgery" reports on his success in saving lives by destroying the "low forms of life" in patients with compound fractures and other wounds, who typically would have died from infection.[58] Carbolic acid is a caustic chemical that kills germs effectively, but also damages human tissues. It has since been replaced by numerous other antiseptics that are less dangerous to people, but still kill microbes. Listerine antiseptic mouthwash, developed by a chemist in 1879, was named for Lister; and although the classic formulation never tasted very good, it does *not* contain the toxic carbolic acid. Its active ingredients are eucalyptol, menthol, methyl salicylate, and thymol, in a solution that contains 27 percent alcohol. The ethyl alcohol is listed as an inactive ingredient, since it is not considered antibacterial at concentrations below 40 percent. Many would argue that 27 percent alcohol (54 proof!) has some activity in the Listerine concoction, which is described and has been advertised as follows: "Sure, it's a little intense, but no other mouthwash can compete with its impressive germ-killing career."[59]

In his work Pasteur had "changed microbes from playthings into useful helpers of mankind," but had not yet revealed the danger of germs, which could be "dread infinitesimal ogres and murdering marauders," causing disease and devastation in the form of epidemics.[60] While many doctors of his day clung to the idea that diseases were caused by bodily humors and atmospheric miasmas (e.g., note that the word *malaria* is Italian for "bad air"), Pasteur doggedly continued to pursue the microscopic basis for many diseases. He and his wife Marie tragically lost three daughters to typhoid fever, and that may have spurred him on his crusade.

Although he was an established and respected scientist, since his ideas were still considered unconventional even Pasteur had an uphill battle to convince the establishment that germs cause disease. His contemporary Robert Koch was a scientific rival, but also an ally in the scientific quest to establish the cause of infectious disease. Through a stepwise approach, known as Koch's postulates, Koch did much difficult groundwork, characterizing microbes and connecting specific germs to specific diseases. Step one is to identify a particular microbe that appears in blood, tissues, mucous, and so on, in every patient or animal with that disease. Step two is to isolate the microorganism from the patient or animal and grow it in the lab, in a pure culture. The third step is to expose a healthy animal to —or inject it with—the microbe, to see if the test subject will become ill. Finally, if the test subject does develop the same disease, isolate the germ from that subject and compare it with the original microbe; if they match, it supports that microbe as the causative agent.[61]

By following Koch's postulates, once a particular germ is shown to cause a disease, it is possible to develop and test cures, such as antibiotics and other antimicrobial drugs, and preventative treatments, such as vaccines. In addition, screening and diagnosis of the disease becomes more feasible. Using this methodology, Koch identified *Bacillus anthracis* as the cause of anthrax in cattle, he discovered various micrococci as the etiology of traumatic infective diseases, and in the culmination of his work he demonstrated that the tubercle bacillus was the causative agent in tuberculosis. The latter was particularly challenging, as this microbe is exceedingly small, grows slowly, and is hard to stain for microscopy. Koch's legacy is in the development of methodologies to isolate and grow microorganisms in the lab so they can be studied and established as causative agents in disease.[62]

Pasteur's legacy continued to grow as he tackled infectious diseases such as anthrax and chicken cholera. In the process of studying the latter, he accidentally discovered how to immunize animals with weakened or attenuated cultures, making the animals resistant to disease. The principle of vaccination had been discovered by Edward Jenner in 1798, when he demonstrated that exposure to cowpox, a much less severe infection in humans, would confer immunity against the disfiguring and highly lethal smallpox virus.[63] Pasteur's contribution was in figuring out that the original microbe itself, if made less active, could confer immunity without much danger to the patient.

Whether it was accidentally or serendipitously, the old cholera cultures Pasteur was using in one experiment failed to make chickens sick; but instead of destroying those chickens and starting over again, he decided to revaccinate the chickens with fresh cholera cultures. Lo and behold, the chickens survived that second challenge, having developed immunity from the first injection of weakened microbes. Pasteur was known to say, "In the field of observation, chance favors only the prepared mind," and his sharp mind was clearly prepared to see what others had overlooked.

Pasteur dramatically and courageously challenged rabies, that disease he had witnessed as a child. In 1886 he applied the principles that he had developed in immunization to save the life of a rabies victim, using a series of inoculations of increasing virulence. His success helped garner support for the founding of the Pasteur Institute, where many prominent scientists have trained and notable discoveries have been made. Pasteur helped establish the germ theory of disease; approaches to immunization against disease; methods to identify, study and counteract germs; and most critically, the importance and use of the scientific method to advance knowledge and improve the quality of life.

Biological Roots of Hygiene
What Are Germs and How Do They Relate to Us?

We share our world with many other species, including a vast number of species of microorganisms, or living creatures that are not visible to the naked eye. On our planet, all the species that have evolved over the course of the last three-and-a-half billion years interact, cooperate, and conflict with each other in dynamic ways that determine how life unfolds for each and every living thing. Humans are part and parcel of the living world, and although we have developed technology to help us survive many of the challenges of living on Earth, we still grapple with our microscopic neighbors that cause disease, the so-called "pathogens." Most of the microscopic world is benign and causes us no harm. For instance, microbes help us produce some of the delightful foods and drinks we enjoy, such as yogurt and alcoholic beverages. Many microbes are beneficial to us and help us survive or enhance our lives, but some microbes pose challenges to our environments, make us sick, or even kill us. There is a tremendous diversity of organisms that carry disease.

Humans tend to categorize everything and attempt to put the world in order, to make it more functional, more symmetrical, or easier to work with. In the home, we might organize the groceries in our kitchen cupboards, lining up similar cans of food, the cereal boxes, and the canisters of sugar and spices. In libraries we organize books according to genre and topic. In the living world, we categorize organisms, or living creatures, according to anatomical structure, cellular organization, and/or genetic properties.

Carl Linnaeus, an eighteenth-century botanist, developed an approach to organizing and categorizing the living world, called the binomial system of nomenclature. Linnaeus published *Systema Naturae*, which classified thousands of plants and animals according to genus and species. Scientists now use International Codes of Nomenclature to organize and classify organisms, from the simplest bacterium, *Mycoplasma genitalium*, all the way up to *Homo sapiens*, human beings. Initially, the living world was simply divided into the plants and the animals. When microbes were first discovered, scientists did not know what to make of them. Yeast, the simple microbe that ferments alcoholic beverages, was originally classified by Cagniard-Latour as a plant.[64]

When microscopes were invented and revealed a whole new world of microorganisms, biologists further classified microbes based on the structures of the cells and on their chemistry, for instance, on how they used energy. In that more sophisticated system of classification, plants continued to be grouped together in the Kingdom Plantae, chiefly based on their ability to use the sun's energy to make sugar. Plants use sunlight energy, carbon dioxide, and water in a process called photosynthesis to produce carbohydrates and oxygen. For instance, an apple tree can convert sunlight, thin air (containing carbon dioxide), and water into an apple, a feat of biochemical magic that humans have yet to replicate.

The Animal Kingdom includes multicelled creatures that consume other living creatures. Animals include a huge diversity of forms, from the lowliest sponges (the brightly colored bowl-like marine creatures that look more like plants than animals) to corals, jellyfish, worms, clams, insects, and all the vertebrates—animals with bones: the fish, reptiles, amphibians, birds, and mammals.

Plants and animals are part of the visible living world, as they are made up of billions to trillions of cells that live and cooperate together as multicellular organisms. An adult human being starts off as a single cell, the fertilized egg, or zygote, and through cell reproduction produces the adult form: trillions of cells that stick together for life, functioning as a single unit—a person—for up to eighty or ninety or one hundred years or more.

Fungi reside in their own kingdom on the basis of how they obtain energy from the environment. Fungi have the ability to reuse energy found in other living forms, by reabsorbing matter from dead organisms. They are the decomposers of our world, and we owe them a great debt, as they repossess and recycle dead material and convert it into other useful forms. In Kingdom Fungi, some of the life forms, such as mushrooms, are visible to the naked eye, and some, such as yeasts, are microscopic. Yeasts found themselves a home in this kingdom based on their metabolism and genetic relationships to other life forms. As we have already discussed, yeasts are beneficial to humans as we take advantage of many biological processes they perform in the food industry. They are used to leaven bread; ferment beer, wine, and whisky; and ripen cheeses.

But some fungi are harmful and cause mucoses, which are fungal diseases affecting the scalp, skin, feet, nails, lungs, or brain. Histoplasmosis and candidiasis are examples of fungal infections found in humans. Some mushrooms are poisonous and produce lethal toxins that can sicken and kill us. Interestingly, some fungal toxins have proven to be of great value to us, thanks to scientists who ingeniously adapted the poisons to make antibiotics, various chemicals that are useful in lab experiments, and other drugs.

The fourth kingdom, Kingdom Protista, includes microscopic single-celled organisms that can live in a wide variety of habitats. Most of them reside side by side with humans without harming us. Marine plankton and algae make up a large population of protists on our planet, and they contribute to a healthy environment by making oxygen and breaking down harmful chemicals. But certain protists pose a hazard, as they are vectors of disease. Species of plasmodia cause malaria, trypanosomes cause African sleeping sickness, and water-based protozoa cause many different types of enterocolitis and diarrheal sicknesses, such as amoebic dysentery.

Next come the bacteria, which used to be classified in one kingdom, Monera. Bacteria differ from other life forms in that their cells, the so-called prokaryotes, are simple in structure. They are missing some of the cell structures found in more complex life forms, the eukaryotes. (Animals, plants, fungi, and protists are eukaryotes.) One prominent difference is that unlike eukaryotes, which have a nucleus where the genes are held, prokaryotes keep their DNA in the main part of the cell, the cytoplasm, together with the other cell materials. Bacteria are smaller than eukaryotes, so they are harder to visualize in the microscope, and they vary in shape, size, how they produce energy, and how they move.

Soon after genetic sequencing became possible in the 1970s, a category of bacteria was discovered that surprised the scientific community. They looked in many ways like the other bacteria, but were dramatically different in regard to their genetic sequence, suggesting that they had diverged from other life forms early on in evolution. They were named the archaea, alluding to their ancient evolutionary origins. Taxonomists, who study and classify life forms, decided to classify archaea separately from all other life forms. With increased knowledge about genetic sequences, taxonomists reclassified many species, reorganizing all species into three domains: eukarya (plants, animals, fungi, and protists), bacteria, and archaea.

Archaea are generally not bacteria we have to worry about, as they are not typically dangerous or pathogenic to humans. The other bacteria are the ones we need to study to understand infectious disease, as they represent the many species that can exploit, infect, and destroy human cells. Tuberculosis, cholera, and anthrax are all caused by bacteria, as are diphtheria, Lyme disease, plague, and tetanus. Research on the life cycle of these microbes helps us to develop new drugs, such as antibiotics, that kill the pathogens but have the fewest side effects on the patient.

In addition to the organisms just described that are made up of living cells, there are other infectious agents that cause disease but are not themselves alive in the strictest sense of the word. These agents, which are not independent creatures, include the viruses, viroids, and prions. Viruses are particles that are made up of genetic material (DNA or RNA) housed in a protective or infectious particle, made of proteins. Some viruses are further enclosed in a viral envelope made up of phospholipids and glycoproteins that the viruses appropriated from their host cells. Viruses carry genetic information and use it to infect and transform living cells. Some viruses infect and hijack host cells, commanding them to produce more viruses. The viral progeny go on to infect other cells. Some viruses infect and alter the way the host cell functions. And some can infect cells and lie dormant for long periods of time, eventually reemerging to strike again.

Viruses are specialized to attack or infect specific types of cells. Some viruses attack only plants, such as the tobacco mosaic virus (TMV), which is the scourge of the tobacco industry. Because it is commercially significant, there has been much research effort and funds directed toward uncovering the mechanisms of TMV infection. Some viruses called bacteriophage, or phage for short, only attack bacteria. Phages have been used as tools to understand many of the basic processes of life, revealing, for instance, how DNA works and how viruses infect cells. Learning about phage can help us understand how to control bacterial processes and possibly develop new approaches to fight pathogenic bacteria.

Viruses that infect animal cells are of the highest concern to us as they can cause human diseases. The influenza virus makes millions of people miserable every year, and from 1976 to 2007, the estimated average death rate from influenza in the United States was more than 23,000 per year.[65] Ebola is a menacing virus, as we have no effective vaccine available, there is no cure, and it is deadly. HIV, which is responsible for AIDS, is also of tremendous concern as scientists have not yet been able to design an effective vaccine. Fortunately, for victims of HIV, we do have antiviral medications that inhibit and interrupt the virus life cycle, thereby extending the lives of many infected people. Some viruses, such as rabies, can cause excruciating pain, suffering, and death, but are fairly uncommon, and thanks to Pasteur are avoidable if treated quickly. Herpes, smallpox, rubella, measles, and mumps are all caused by viruses; but since we have developed vaccines for these diseases, we can diminish the risk of those diseases in the population through vaccination programs. In developed countries where vaccination is routine, most people are at low risk for those viral diseases, but in developing countries many still become sick and die from preventable diseases.

Viroids are tiny infectious pathogens, made up of only a small piece of RNA, with no protein coat. They most frequently cause diseases in plants. Potato spindle tuber viroid can lead to slower sprouting and smaller leaves on infected potato or tomato plants.

Prions are infectious particles made of only proteins, and although they have no genetic material (DNA or RNA) they can infect the brains of animals, including humans, leading to neurodegenerative disease. An infected brain develops holes like a sponge, affecting brain function. Prions can be transmitted from one individual to another, but this is quite rare, as it requires direct contact with infected tissues from a victim. A human form of the disease, Kuru, found in New Guinea, appears to be transmitted via ritual cannibalism, through the ingestion of the brain or spinal cords of infected humans. There have been cases of mad cow disease being transmitted from cows to humans, particularly in Great Britain, but they also are rare and appear to be caused by the consumption of meat from infected cattle. Most of us will never encounter disease-causing prions, but it is useful to know that we should avoid eating the brains of infected people or animals.

The greatest medical triumph with regard to viral diseases has been the successful campaign against smallpox and, to a lesser degree, polio. Through worldwide vaccination, smallpox has essentially been eradicated from our planet. The war against polio likewise has been a success story, although pockets of polio cases do still appear, mostly in corners of the world that are not yet developed, or that resist modern health practices for religious or political reasons. The United States was also on the road to eradicating childhood diseases such as measles, mumps, and rubella, but an unfounded and unscientific movement has hampered the success. The antivaccination movement is based on the incorrect notion that vaccines can cause autism. This is wholly unsupported by scientific research, which unequivocally shows no relation between childhood vaccinations and autism. Unfortunately, this misguided movement has led to innocent victims, mostly children, contracting unnecessary and hazardous diseases.

Life forms on Earth interact with each other, sometimes cooperatively, sometimes destructively, sometimes predictably, and sometimes erratically. When considering infectious diseases, it is important to understand how organisms have evolved over billions of years, side by side, like members of a very large and sometimes dysfunctional family. Just as in a human family there can be cooperative, exploitative, and destructive relationships, in the worldwide family of living things there are interdependent, symbiotic relationships, which include: mutualism, or cooperative relationships; commensalism, which are neutral or exploitative relationships; and parasitism, or destructive relationships. The latter, parasitism, and pathogenesis are those relationships that cause harm to one party in particular.

Examples of mutualism and cooperation are the bacteria of the human gut that produce vitamins B and K and help us to digest certain food molecules. In return, those bacteria are provided with a warm incubator, our gut, and plenty of nutrients for their growth and reproduction. Commensalism is when one organism benefits and the other is neither harmed nor helped. The bacteria on our hands hang out on our skin, hitching a ride, neither harming nor benefitting us. (In truth, we do benefit indirectly, as the harmless bacteria fill a void and crowd out or compete with disease-causing bacteria.) When the relationship is parasitic, one species benefits and the other is harmed. Pathogenic, disease-causing microbes have that negative relationship with their hosts, whether the hosts are humans, other animals, plants, or other microbes.

Microorganisms in our environment have complex relationships with humans: Some are beneficial, some are neutral, and some cause harm to human beings. So when we talk about managing microbes in our environment, it is important to specify which ones we are addressing. We do not want to eliminate the microbes that are part of our normal flora—the microbes that reside in and on healthy bodies and contribute to a healthy existence. We do want to avoid germs that can infect, produce toxins, or compete with the microflora that keep us healthy.

We take it for granted that when we catch contagious diseases there are reliable treatments available. They are based on the past two hundred years of discoveries by courageous scientists with prepared minds, such as Pasteur and Semmelweis, who had the insight to discover the nature of infections. It is frustrating when uneducated people reject basic health principles and basic hygiene, but it is even more disturbing when members of the educated public reject scientific knowledge and empirical proof, challenging, for instance, the use of vaccines, even though the scientific evidence for their value is convincing. But people will believe all sorts of unscientific tales, including the "Five-Second Rule" (see chapter 4).

From what we have learned in the past two centuries, we know that many microbes can be blamed for disease and death, and there are proven ways we can avoid being infected by them. Semmelweis, Pasteur, Lister, and others were heroes for humanity, and their scientific ideas prevail. When humans began to take the advice of the microbe hunters, they started to live longer, healthier lives. For this the pioneers of hygiene deserve our respect and gratitude.

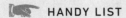 HANDY LIST

The Most Important Hygiene Developments in Human History

1 Ritual washing: Different cultures and religions have ritual washing procedures that go back hundreds and even thousands of years, whose goals are primarily ritual purity, not hygiene. Washing rituals, even when done without cleansers, can be effective in reducing the risk of disease and improving health. (Although in some cases they can do the opposite—some ritual washing practices can spread disease among the populations.)

2 Unconventional methods of hand hygiene, that is, dry ablution, with mud, ash, sand, or dust, may reduce the risk of infectious disease.

3 Infrastructure, including public baths, waste management, and wells: These technologies and developments were not restricted to modern times. In ancient societies they also contributed to healthier communities. Accessible clean water is essential to the health of communities.

4 Microbes are everywhere: Scientific research documenting the presence of animalcules in rainwater, between teeth, and virtually everywhere set the stage for the discovery of disease-causing organisms. (Leeuwenhoek)

5 Disproving spontaneous generation: Proving that all life comes from preexisting life helped us to understand how disease is spread and how to disinfect the environment and protect ourselves. (Spallanzani, Pasteur)

6 Infectious diseases are caused by microbes: Demonstrating the germ theory of disease was essential for learning how to diagnose and control transmission of disease. (Fracastoro, Lister, Koch, Pasteur)

7 Handwashing reduces the spread and incidence of infectious disease: This notion led to immediate solutions and improvements in medical practice; however, it was not widely accepted, and it was even actively rejected for some time. (Semmelweis, Lister)

8 Vaccination strategies and solutions: Developed with the insight of Pasteur and Jenner, immunizations helped to conquer numerous infectious diseases. (Pasteur, Jenner, others)

9 Disease-causing microorganisms can be fungi, bacteria, viruses, or prions: This knowledge and the ability to study the genes of infectious microbes has advanced the field and holds tremendous promise for eradicating much disease and suffering in the future.

First Do No Harm

Thanks to improved nutrition and hygiene, as well as the development of antibiotics and vaccinations, there has been a dramatic increase in average life expectancy in the last hundred years. According to the Centers for Disease Control and Prevention (CDC) statistics, a baby born at the turn of the twentieth century had a life expectancy of 47.3 years. In the early 1900s, infant mortality was high, women routinely died in childbirth, and tuberculosis and other infectious diseases were common and typically fatal. A little more than a century later, the life expectancy for a baby born in the United States in 2012 is close to 79.8 years. What a difference a century of medical advances makes. While this increase in life expectancy is impressive, it is disappointing that world health statistics rank the United States thirty-sixth in the world for life expectancy, behind much of Europe, Australia (no. 9), Canada (no. 11), Israel (no. 13), Taiwan (no. 31), and Japan (no. 1).[1] There is room for improvement in U.S. health and medical care.

Routine handwashing and other hygienic practices have helped us achieve dramatic improvements in health and have extended life expectancy. We are well aware of the causes of infectious diseases and how to reduce risks. Thus it is shocking that a patient who enters a hospital for surgery, or a routine procedure, can be exposed to and sometimes contract a serious life-threatening infectious disease. We should do all we can to reduce and try to eliminate this threat.

Many medical institutions work hard and devote significant resources to reducing the spread of infectious diseases. They know how nosocomial, that is, hospital-acquired infections, occur and how to reduce the risk of these diseases. But when people are involved, careless errors and lackadaisical attitudes about hand hygiene can lead to the spread of disease.

A few years ago I was rushed to a local emergency room because of severe abdominal pain. In the course of my stay, diagnosis, and treatment for an umbilical hernia, I noticed that there was only one functioning sink in the emergency room; it happened to be situated near my bed. There were a few other sinks in the facility, which apparently were not working. The staff working in other parts of the facility had to walk quite a distance to wash their hands. Since I was lying around for some time waiting for tests and treatment, I had the opportunity to observe the use of the sink. In the course of the seven or so hours I was there, I noticed that not many of the medical personnel made the effort to use the lone functioning sink. My conclusion was that few of the staff washed their hands on a regular basis.

On another occasion I was admitted to the hospital for acute back pain and was to receive an injection of hydrocortisone into my spine. I observed the nurse peel open the sterile packaging of the needle, and the needle fell to the floor. I asked her to open a new one for me. She promptly drew the curtains around my bed so that I would not be able to watch her anymore. I don't know whether she used a fresh instrument for my procedure. (Does the Five-Second Rule apply in hospitals? The Five-Second Rule is the unfounded and unscientific notion that food that falls on the floor can still be used if it is recovered within five seconds. Many otherwise rational people follow that practice. We hope healthcare professionals do not.)

These anecdotal accounts of my own experiences in two separate hospitals, in two different states, are admittedly a very small sample of experiences. (I should note here that the outcomes of my hospital treatments were positive, and that I recovered nicely from my ailments.) But a broader survey of practices in hospitals and other medical personnel confirms my impression from my own experiences and shows that consistent hand hygiene is far from universal and not scrupulously followed.

Standard of Care/Best Practice

The worst-case scenario in medical practice is when a patient develops complications, the patient's condition worsens, or worst of all, dies, as a result of the medical intervention. Therefore "first do no harm" is a prime directive of bioethics. In the spirit of helping and not harming, protocols and practices have been developed in all areas of medicine to establish the minimum-accepted levels of performance. In medicine these guidelines are known as "standard of care," or best practice.[2]

The "standard of care" can refer to the process used to diagnose and treat patients, as long as it conforms to the accepted practices of the profession and meets or exceeds a certain level of medical expertise. The proper treatment for particular diseases and conditions, or "best practice," may vary depending on the patient, the illness, the prognosis, and even the available resources. Standard of care in a major medical center will differ from that in a MASH unit near the front lines of battle. The legal definition of the phrase refers to a level of care that responsible and similarly qualified medical practitioners in a particular community would provide for similar cases, hence differences may arise from community to community and in clinics of varied resources. In order to demonstrate medical malpractice in a lawsuit, it is necessary to prove that the physician has failed to perform at that appropriate standard of care widely used by medical practitioners.[3] When a chiropractor injured my back some years ago, I was advised that it would be difficult to demonstrate malpractice since he was doing what was appropriate for chiropractic practice, that is, manipulating the spine. I suffered greatly with a ruptured disk, but had no recourse other than to campaign vociferously against chiropractic medicine, which I learned can be hazardous to your health.

Why should we care about standard of care? Because the medical community cares enough to establish standards, and treatment that does not rise to those standards can lead to calamitous results. As already discussed, my mother entered the hospital for a cardiovascular condition, but her surgery and other medical procedures led to infections. As the infection spread through her already frail body and overwhelmed her immune system, critical systems were compromised and began to fail. After almost six months in the intensive care unit (ICU) struggling valiantly to recover, she succumbed to the complications. To be sure, this is not an indictment of the medical profession, rather it is a call for vigilance with regard to standard of care, and a plea to continually strive to raise those standards and not be complacent.

The Principles of Bioethics

Primum non nocere, or "first do no harm," has been the first and foremost expectation of medical personnel for thousands of years and a major principle of bioethics. This concept has roots in the Oath of Hippocrates, the pledge of medical practitioners, written some twenty-five hundred years ago. Bioethics principles of more recent vintage emerged after World War II, when atrocities performed by Nazi doctors were exposed and documented. During the Holocaust, which spanned from 1933 to 1945, the Nazis systematically and deliberately misused and corrupted medicine and science. Among their abuses, they forced concentration camp prisoners to serve as subjects of tortuous, agonizing, and lethal experiments. After the war, the Nuremberg trials of Nazi perpetrators, including Nazi doctors and nurses, exposed the violations of medical ethics and led to development of the Nuremberg Code, a formal statement of principles regarding patient care and the treatment of research subjects. A major tenet of the Nuremberg Code is that "the voluntary consent of the human subject is absolutely essential."[4]

Among the prominent ethicists, philosophers, and scientists of the modern era who have addressed the issues of ethics in medical care, Tom Beauchamp and James Childress stand out. They articulated four principles of modern bioethics that stand as cornerstones of the discipline. Two of the four principles, *nonmaleficence* (do no harm) and *beneficence* (do good) are rooted in the ancient tradition established by disciples of Hippocrates. The other two principles, namely autonomy and justice, also aim to protect patients and human research subjects. *Autonomy* refers to the patient's right to determine the level of medical care he or she desires, and *justice* can be understood as the fair and equitable access to medical care and other resources. All four principles, and related ethical guidelines, influence our modern medical system, resulting in a "standard of care" for proper treatment that includes the utilization of "best practices."[5]

The field of bioethics has developed rapidly in recent years. More than ten years ago, when I developed my university's first workshops, and then a formal course in bioethics, there were few such courses in existence and few textbooks in the field. Today many universities and medical facilities offer courses and training on bioethics and medical ethics issues, and there are dozens of textbooks to choose from. Now there are graduate and certification programs in bioethics; it has evolved into a formal discipline of its own. The growth spurt in this new field is likely because of the explosion of technology in medical practice: technology that extends and redefines the end of life, technology that enables previously sterile couples to conceive, and technology that enables the screening for and selection of genetic traits. Bioethics is a modern discipline that melds aspects of biology, health care, research, the environment, religion, philosophy, ethics, and the law.

From the perspective of medical hygiene, a basic expectation since Semmelweis, Lister, Pasteur, and Koch discovered the causes of infectious disease and contagion (chapter 2) is that physicians, nurses, and others who tend to patients should wash their hands. It is part of the expectation of "best practices" and a "standard of care" in medicine. Medical personnel must wash their hands before patient contact to protect the patient and after patient contact to protect themselves and other patients. The simple procedure of handwashing dramatically reduces risk and saves lives.

Bad hygiene kills people. Doctors, nurses, and other trained medical professionals, who should know better, do not always scrupulously follow best practices with regard to hygiene, including handwashing. The prime directive of medical ethics is "first do no harm." On one hand, the bioethics principle of nonmaleficence, that the action of the physician should not harm the patient, is contradicted when doctors and nurses fail to wash their hands, putting patients at risk. On the other hand, the bioethics principle of beneficence, that is, all actions should be for the benefit of the patient, is supported by medical professionals who do conscientiously wash their hands.

Most healthcare professionals are dedicated to performing their duties to the best of their abilities, with the goal of healing patients and improving their outcomes. That said, all medical personnel are human, and mistakes, errors, and omissions occur, sometimes leading to disaster and the death of the patient. Gloves break and instruments drop. Doctors and nurses may need to rush from patient to patient and in the process make mistakes. The old saying, "haste makes waste," is no nursery rhyme. It is a serious declaration of caution, as haste may lead to careless errors, and medical errors lead to serious complications and even death. It has been estimated that four hundred thousand deaths per year in the United States can be attributed to medical errors.[6] And hospital-acquired infections account for tens of thousands of U.S. deaths per year.[7] Nosocomial, or hospital-acquired infections, are serious life threats due to drug-resistant strains such as MRSA, which are notoriously hard to combat. Now multi-drug resistance has resulted in bacterial infections that do not respond to treatment. Varying from year to year, some sources estimate that in the United States alone, 5 to 10 percent of hospitalized patients are affected, translating to two million patients, ninety thousand deaths, and a cost of $5 billion per year.[8] Anything we can do to reduce the risk of hospital-acquired infection is worth the effort.

Worldwide figures on medical errors and nosocomial infections are more complicated to calculate, as many countries cannot provide the standard of medical care we enjoy in the United States, and many areas of the world do not formally monitor statistics on healthcare outcomes. As we saw from the Ebola epidemic, the standard of care for Ebola in the United States is high, leading to a better outcome for patients here than in the African nations where the spread of disease is rampant and upward of 70 percent of victims died. We should not rest on our laurels though, as there are numerous other countries with better outcomes than the United States. We lag behind in infant mortality rates and average life expectancy, and we can do better to improve our "best practices." According to the U.S. Department of Health and Human Services, in 2013 the United States ranked twenty-seventh among industrialized nations (among countries with over 2.5 million population) for infant mortality, and as previously mentioned, we ranked thirty-sixth for average life expectancy in 2012.[9]

Hand Hygiene in the Operating Room

The preparation required to perform surgery is comprehensive and complicated. Thanks to Lister, Semmelweis, and others, doctors and nurses follow strict protocols in order to reduce the risk of outside contamination in the operating room. After all, if surgery is involved, the skin, our primary protection from the external environment, is being breached. In many cases, patients already have wounds and other breaches that have been exposed to infectious agents and may already be contaminated, carrying microorganisms that put the patient at risk. The operating room is not an entirely sterile environment, but the procedures used in the OR are designed to minimize exposure and risk of infection.

Although there are accepted protocols for scrubbing and gloving for surgery, there is some disagreement on methodology. Surgical hand-washing is an art unto itself. When my father washed his hands before eating, sometimes he would humorously hold his cleansed arms fingers up, palms toward his face, and elbows down, mimicking the posture of surgeons who had just scrubbed. He did it with an amused expression, as he was not a surgeon, but he "played one at home." (In a well-known 1984 TV commercial the actor says, "I'm not a doctor but I play one on TV," and then goes on to recommend cough syrup for adults.)[10]

The protocol for preoperative scrubbing varies. For many years a minimum of ten minutes of scrubbing was expected. Now there are numerous variations on the theme. What all preoperative scrubbing has in common is the goal of reducing the contamination on the surface of the hands before donning the sterile gown and gloves. The hands themselves, although cleansed and decontaminated, are never completely germfree (sterile) after scrubbing.

At Cedars-Sinai Medical Center in Los Angeles, the operating room guidelines for surgical hand scrub procedure recommends a "thorough washing, rinsing, and drying of hands and arms at the beginning of the day or if skin is visibly contaminated."[11] The antisepsis procedure follows the Association of Operating Room Nursing (AORN) practices and standards. Surgical staff first inspect the skin of the hands for lesions (open cuts, abrasions, etc.), which could increase the likelihood of contamination. All artificial fingernail enhancements (tips, acrylics) and all rings, watches, and bracelets must be removed. A scrub sink is used that has a special faucet for handless operation, or handles that can be operated using elbows or foot pedals. Hands are first rinsed, then basic handwashing with soap and water is done up to two inches above the elbows. The surgical sponge package is opened. Each package has a sterile sponge impregnated with cleanser (hexachlorophene, povidone-iodine, or chlorhexidine) and a sterile nail pick. The nail pick is used to remove dirt from under the nails, then discarded. The disposable scrub brush with antimicrobial agent is used to scrub the hands and forearms either by timing (three minutes) or by brush-stroke count. For the brush-stroke method, the scrub brush is wetted with water and used for thirty strokes on nails and fingertips and repeated for other hand. The brush is wetted with water again, as needed, and used in a deliberate way to scrub every surface of each finger (four surfaces per finger) ten times. The interdigitary webbed surfaces between fingers are also scrubbed. Hands are scrubbed for ten strokes to each of the four hand surfaces, and the process is repeated for the other fingers and hand. Then scrubbing continues with ten strokes to each of the four arm surfaces, and repeated for the other arm. Timed scrubbing is forty-five seconds for each hand and forty-five seconds for each arm. "If you accidentally contaminate an area, you must rescrub it."[12] When finished, the brush is dropped into a trash receptacle. Rinsing is done with running water from elevated fingertips downward toward palms, wrists, and arms to elbows, always in order from most sterile (hands) to least sterile (elbows). The dripping wet arms must be held with fingertips up and elbows down, so that the water drips down toward the elbows, and not the reverse. Otherwise, contaminants from the elbows can drip onto the hands. It is important once the handwashing is done not to touch any surface that is not sterile. A sterile towel is used to blot dry fingertips, palms, back of hands, wrists, arms, and elbows, in that order. The sterile gown is donned and "closed gloving" is used to pull gloves on over the sterile sleeves of the gown. Finally, the fingers are inserted into the sterile gloves. If there is any breach, or the sterile surfaces contact a nonsterile surface, the scrubbing starts again.

Although many surgeons still follow traditional scrubbing methods, thanks to empirical research in many hospitals, including Cedars-Sinai, the scrubless-waterless-brushless skin preparation may be used. Hands need to start off clean and dry. Two ml of Avagard (3M Corp, containing 1 percent chlorhexidine gluconate and 61 percent ethyl alcohol, along with moisturizers) is dispensed into one cupped palm. The fingertips of the other hand are dipped into the hand-wash solution, and it is worked under the nails and over all surfaces of the hand, wrist, arm, and just above the elbow. The procedure is repeated on the other hand. A second round is completed, applying hand wash to both hands up to the wrist. Hands are allowed to air dry before donning the gown and gloves.

Reflecting research that shows no significant increase in contamination, the duration of the scrubbing protocol has been reduced from a ten-minute scrub, to a three-minute one. An Austrian study reports that "mode and duration of the treatment have significantly changed over time."[13] In that paper, Suchomel and coauthors reported that alcohol-based hand rubs have been used for over a hundred years in Europe and are finally be-coming more accepted in North America as well. A French study compar-ing alcohol-based hand rubs with traditional methods of hand scrubbing concluded that their alcoholic hand-rubbing procedure "was as effective as traditional hand-scrubbing with antiseptic soap in preventing surgical site infections."[14]

The question of whether handwashing or hand rubs are better at disin-fection continues to be studied. Although not strictly an operating room, a dermatologist's office is a medical facility where minor surgical proce-dures are performed and patients with complex skin lesions are treated. Hence, there is a strong emphasis on best practices in hygiene. One re-search article, entitled, "Hand Hygiene in the Dermatologist's Office: To Wash or to Rub?" concludes that "ABHRs [alcohol-based hand rubs] are preferred over standard hand washing with soap and water and should serve as a primary mode of hand disinfection in dermatology offices."[15] They recommend handwashing with antiseptic soap "after restroom, be-fore eating, and when hands are visibly soiled by blood or bodily fluids."[16] Other times alcohol-based hand rubs can suffice, and are even preferred, because of their ease of use, accessibility, overall compliance, effective-ness in killing many types of germs, and reduction of incidence of hand dermatitis. Nowadays many alcohol-based hand rubs are less irritating than antiseptic hand washes. In dermatologists' offices this is important, as many procedures involve minor surgery and skin lesions that are highly susceptible to infection, and medical staff have to sanitize their hands multiple times per day. Messina and coworkers do report that alcohol rubs are not effective against the perilous germ *Clostridium difficile*, and they recommend handwashing in clinical situations where infection with that bacterium is a risk. In addition, "Wear gloves and use other barrier devices when procedures are performed or clinical site contains known infectious materials."[17] Regardless of the details of preoperative or clinical cleans-ing, the goal is to be as close to germfree as possible, when operating on or treating patients.

In addition to hand hygiene for medical practitioners, the patients' skin also must be sanitized before surgery by using antiseptics, as their skin and wounds can be a source of dangerous microbes. Before certain pro-cedures, patients are given special soap, such as chlorhexidine gluconate (or CHG, used at Beth Israel Deaconess Medical Center of Harvard Medical School) and instructed to wash their body with this antiseptic soap, with particular attention to the surgical area, before arriving at the hospital. In the OR immediately before the operation, the skin area to be operated on is scrubbed with iodophore, an iodine-containing product with antiseptic activity, and then painted with iodine solution, to reduce or eliminate bacteria, viruses, and other microbes.

Alternative ways to prepare the patient's skin were tested in a study that compared three skin preparation methods: iodophore scrub for three minutes, followed by painting the skin with povidone-iodine; iodophore scrub for five minutes, followed by painting the skin; and painting alone. The conclusion was that painting alone with povidone-iodine can be used for preoperative skin preparation since the additional step of iodine scrubbing does not improve the outcome.[18] This type of research study may not sound dramatic, but the small changes built on scientific observations and testing can lead to an improved standard of care and better outcomes for patients.

Compliance
Increasing Handwashing by Healthcare Workers

As we have learned from the Ebola scare, swine-flu outbreaks, and myriad other diseases, the medical community and media continue to remind us that handwashing can serve as the first barrier against transmission of disease from person to person. Apparently not all medical professionals practice what is preached.

This is a serious problem because nosocomial, or hospital-acquired infections, pose a significant threat to patients who are already sick. Those types of infections occur when patients are exposed to germs from other patients or medical personnel. Patients being treated for one disease or condition can get sicker if they contract illnesses from unsanitized equipment or materials, solutions, hands, or other sources of contact. Nosocomial infections can occur in hospitals, clinics, or other healthcare facilities and can sicken and kill thousands of people every year. Such infections are particularly difficult to treat because the types of germs that occur in hospitals are frequently resistant to antibiotics. Ironically, the overuse of antibiotics has contributed considerably to this problem, as this has helped to generate and encourage the growth of strains of bacteria that are harder and harder to eradicate. The infections that result can have serious consequences and complications, and even cause the death of the patient.

Poor hand hygiene is a significant risk factor, and improvement in compliance does save lives. The importance of handwashing was well established in a study of very low birth-weight infants. In one hospital in Bologna, Italy, after the neonatal intensive care unit (ICU) instituted a standardized hand-hygiene program, including washing with antimicrobial soap and the use of alcohol-based hand gels, the rate of nosocomial infections was reduced from 16.6 percent to 5.8 percent in premature infants. Reducing the risk of such complications in the tiniest of patients undoubtedly saved those very new lives.[19]

At a Tennessee hospital, a survey of healthcare workers (HCW) showed that mean adherence to hand hygiene in all ICUs was 54 percent, meaning that almost half the time workers failed to wash their hands. There was a dramatic difference in handwashing in adult ICUs (35 percent) versus pediatric ICUs (90 percent). Why did personnel do so much better in the pediatric ICUs? Attitude, education, and supervision may have played a role in performance in the pediatric wards. After interventions were implemented, there was a dramatic and significant improvement in hand-hygiene adherence in adult ICUs (81 percent).[20] (Pediatric ICUs were not significantly changed, but they started off very high.)

In that Tennessee hospital it was also learned that hospital workers were not well educated regarding the use of alcohol-based hand-rub solutions. Almost half believed that the alcohol solutions would not work for methicillin-resistant *Staphylococcus aureus* (MRSA) infections, and 21 percent thought that hand-rub solutions could be used if hands were soiled. In fact, alcohol-based hand rubs are effective against MRSA, but hands need to be washed with soap and water if they are dirty. Alcohol-based hand rubs may kill germs, but they don't clean dirt off hands. "The survey of HCWs revealed gaps in knowledge regarding methods of hand hygiene," concludes the article.[21]

Studies show that doctors have a worse record in handwashing than nurses and other medical professionals. A 2008 study at a Toledo hospital revealed an inverse relationship between the level of professional medical education and rate of handwashing compliance. That is to say, medical attending physicians were significantly less likely to wash their hands than nurses. Furthermore, doctors were less likely to improve their behavior in response to intervention. After a visit of the Joint Commission on Accreditation of Healthcare Organizations (JCAHO) to the hospital, nurses improved their handwashing compliance but doctors did not.[22] Is there any way we can get through to physicians that they need to place more attention on their own hand hygiene? How can we motivate doctors to improve with regard to handwashing?

Messina and coauthors highlighted positive and negative factors associated with hand-hygiene compliance. Positive factors include: a clinical site with a high risk of transferring disease-causing pathogens; cleansing agents conveniently located and including better-tolerated antiseptics; medical staff who understood the advantages of alcohol-based hand rubs (ABHR) over handwashing, as well as the benefit for the patients; being a nurse; and being female. Negative factors include: a low risk of patients infecting medical personnel; inconvenient hand-hygiene facilities; working in a busy and high-stress environment where there is insufficient time; being a doctor; and being male.[23]

What factors among these lists can be addressed in order to improve hand hygiene? Even though several research studies demonstrate that female nurses do better on compliance, it would be impractical, and discriminatory, to suggest that only female nurses and doctors have contact with patients. The hustle and bustle of busy clinics and wards is unlikely to be changed anytime soon. More pragmatic approaches would be redesigning wards to include convenient sinks and alcohol hand-rub stations, and educating personnel regarding the risks and benefits of best practices in hygiene.

"When in Doubt, Throw It Out"

If my own experiences and those of many others (see following) are representative of common hospital practice, it is easy to understand how infections spread in hospitals. In order to maintain sterility and not transmit germs from one source to another, there are specific practices that can be followed. For many years I conducted cell culture research projects that required aseptic technique. *Aseptic technique* refers to lab and clinical practices that maintain a germfree environment. In clinical work, it involves implementing procedures to protect patients from infectious agents during surgery or other high-risk activities.

I worked on a number of research projects involving cell culture, where cells that have been removed from animals are grown in culture dishes. In this procedure, the cells have to be kept entirely germfree; it is imperative to keep all bacteria, viruses, and fungi from infecting the culture vessel and attacking the cells. If the cells become contaminated, they could die from the infection. Even if they survive the infection, they will still harbor the microorganisms, and the presence of the contaminating microbes will interfere with the results of the studies or interpretation of data. For instance, if a scientist wants to study how cells react to a drug, microorganisms in the culture could also metabolize and alter the drug, confounding the results of the experiment.

In the 1980s during the early days of in vitro fertilization, I worked as the embryologist in an infertility clinic, making test-tube babies. The new technology was in its infancy (no pun intended). We designed and set up the first in vitro fertilization laboratory in New York State, at Mount Sinai Medical Center. We learned from in vitro pioneers at the Jones Institute in Virginia how to prepare the sperm and eggs, how to fertilize and cultivate the embryos, and best practices to keep them from becoming contaminated in their petri dishes in the incubator. It was critical to maintain aseptic conditions; the success of the procedure was at stake. Sterility was essential to the success of the procedure—the human embryos were dependent on an obsessive attention to keeping them free of contamination.

Germfree conditions can be maintained if certain rules are consistently followed, and contaminations can be minimized if careful techniques are employed. For instance, to prevent microbes from entering an open bottle or other vessel, whenever the bottle is opened, it should be done in an enclosed environment. Any procedures involving the transfer of liquids or the movement of an egg or embryo from one vessel to another is typically performed in a laminar flow hood, which is an enclosed environment with controlled airflow. Laminar flow hoods have fans and filters that produce an air screen. They are designed to reduce the chance that germs from the outside, including those from the scientist or physician, are transferred through the air into the sterile, experimental vessels.

It is also necessary to ensure that the nutrient media or supplies such as petri dishes, flasks, and pipets, are presterilized. Liquids, metals, and glass materials can be sterilized by autoclave—a steam and high-pressure system that kills bacteria, viruses, and other microbes. Disposable plastic-ware is purchased presterilized and packaged. Since plastic items would melt if exposed to high temperatures, they are sterilized by the manufacturers using radiation or toxic gas.

Packaged liquids and materials are opened only under a laminar flow hood, or in a sterile field of an operating room or clinic. Once open, they can become contaminated from the air, or by touching hands or other surfaces. For instance, the needle that fell on the floor during my procedure would have become contaminated from whatever dirt and germs were on the floor. Once an instrument is opened, it will no longer be sterile if it contacts anything that harbors microbes. A good rule of thumb that I use when doing cell or embryo culture is: "when in doubt, throw it out." In other words, if you think that something has been contaminated, then do not use it for an experiment or, even more critically, a patient. It is short-sighted to risk using a possibly contaminated item on a patient, whose health may be compromised. Some items can be set aside to be resterilized and reused at a later time. But disposable materials that are contaminated must be discarded. While this appears to be wasteful, it is, in fact, the wisest course, as it reduces the chance of later complications associated with infection and disease.

I recently saw a commercial on television for presterilized catheters. A catheter is a tube that is inserted from outside the body, through the urethra, and into the urinary bladder to facilitate urination. The actor in the advertisement is bemoaning the fact that she has to reuse her catheters, and she needs to cleanse and boil her catheters every time she reuses them. Unsanitized catheters can introduce germs into the bladder, leading to bladder infections and possibly even kidney infections. The advertisement for disposable, one-use presterilized catheters claims that use of their product will reduce the risk of infections. This commercial correctly emphasized the importance of sterility for patient health. (It also reaffirmed the notion that "anything goes" on TV today. There are, apparently, no boundaries with regard to what is discussed in ads. Incontinence, impotence, contraception, diarrhea, constipation, and now catheterization are all topics for TV—especially around dinnertime.)

When working in the lab or clinic, it may be tempting to use materials that might have become contaminated, or have been exposed to contamination, because the items are expensive, or it would be inconvenient (or impossible) to get a replacement. But that practice is risky. Taking shortcuts in aseptic technique in a research lab could jeopardize the hours, weeks, months, and sometimes even years of preparation done for a particular experiment. More critical yet, is that cutting corners in clinical situations could jeopardize the health and well-being of patients. Taking shortcuts for tissue culture or patient care is never justified, even if it means extra expense or delaying a procedure until the sterile materials are available.

Many doctors and nurses are proficient in the practice of aseptic technique. Most are aware of the elaborate procedures used in operating rooms. We see the scrubbing, gloving, and gowning of surgeons and maintenance of highly sanitized operating rooms on television medical dramas such as *Grey's Anatomy* and comedies such as *Scrubs*. However, even in those environments and under the best conditions, mistakes can be made and corners may be cut. Patients can become infected from germs entering open wounds or being introduced into the body through unsterile catheters, needles, solutions, or flawed procedures. For instance, a biopsy that is intended to be diagnostic (breast, prostate, skin) can become infected and lead to serious medical complications. In a study of Canadian men undergoing prostate biopsy, the overall risk of hospitalization due to infection was 1.9 percent,[24] which is almost one in fifty.

In more routine procedures, for instance, those performed in doctors', dentists', or other clinical offices, there may be even less adherence to sterile technique than found in surgery suites and ORs. Doctors' offices do not have all the facilities of a fully stocked hospital or an operating room. They may or may not have access to a sterilizer. It may not be possible to maintain very strict standards of aseptic technique. But even in those settings, there are compelling reasons to scrupulously maintain aseptic technique. The health and life of a patient may depend on it.

Wherever a medical procedure is performed, hygienic techniques are only effective if the personnel are trained and are willing to follow protocol. Doctors, nurses, and other medical professionals may not be sufficiently educated in every aspect of hygiene, or they may forget to follow procedures. As seen in television medical dramas, and in real life, doctors and nurses may be overworked and rushing through a procedure, or rushing from one patient to another. Sometimes workers are trying to conserve resources and hesitate to discard material or supplies that might have been exposed to contamination.

Just as I do in my lab, when dealing with food in my own kitchen, I subscribe to the philosophy "when in doubt throw it out." That is to say, if I think that something might have spoiled, I choose to discard it rather than take a chance of an upset stomach or food poisoning. I have always applied this principle to my tissue culture and in vitro fertilization work, as mentioned prior, and have rarely experienced contaminated cultures. Best practices in medicine call for scrupulous adherence to hygienic techniques, including the use of sterile instruments and careful handwashing. If there is any doubt about sterility, the equipment should be discarded or resterilized, even if it increases costs or takes more time.

A Worldwide Problem

Old habits die hard. In nursing and medical school there is an emphasis on sterile technique, but there is cause for concern about what happens once doctors and nurses begin to practice. And it is a worldwide problem, particularly problematic in some countries, so if you can help it, don't get sick while traveling.

A study in a Spanish teaching hospital revealed that "although hand hygiene is the most important measure in the prevention of nosocomial infection, adherence to recommendations among health care workers (HCW) is low."[25] This study was performed by direct observation of handwashing by healthcare workers. Mean compliance was a paltry 20 percent, although the level of compliance varied according to the area of the hospital studied. For instance, in the intensive care unit compliance was 69 percent, while in surgical wards the figure was 4.3 percent. These numbers are shocking, since patients in the ICU are recovering from serious illness, they are very frail, and they are prone to infection. More disturbing yet is that handwashing rates were twice as frequent after contact with patients

(25.6 percent) as compared with handwashing before contact with patients (12.8 percent).[26] That suggests that hospital personnel were more concerned with protecting themselves than they were with protecting their patients from nosocomial infections.

Healthcare workers who were studied in a hospital in Riyadh, Saudi Arabia, had a 6.7 percent frequency of handwashing before patient contact and 23.7 percent after patient contact. While medical students and interns washed hands about 70 percent of the time, the handwashing frequency for nurses was only 18.8 percent, for residents 12.5 percent, and for consultants 9.1 percent. When hands were washed, they were not washed adequately, with the duration of washing averaging 4.7 seconds per incident. Glove wearing was observed an average of 75.5 percent of the time. "Poor adherence to handwashing is a worldwide problem," conclude the authors.[27]

In the most recent experience with Ebola and past episodes of the so-called "swine flu" (H1N1), we learned that not only can the spread of disease be rampant, but epidemics can be particularly disastrous in communities lacking the most basic resources, such as clean water. In the Mexican healthcare system, as in other developing countries, the lack of basic amenities contributes to the problem of poor hygiene in hospitals.

A public general hospital in San Luis Potosi, Mexico, was the site of a study on nosocomial infections in children under the age of fifteen. Over the course of fifteen years, the hospital implemented various interventions to improve compliance in handwashing, to reduce the overcrowding of wards, and to establish improved handling of catheters and intravenous solutions. For instance, the use of a laminar flow hood was introduced for the preparation of intravenous solutions. The rate of nosocomial infections in children did decrease, although the mortality rate of children who were infected was still high (45.2 percent of children with gram-negative bacterial bloodstream infection and 19.2 percent of children with gram-positive bacterial infection died); but interventions and education can improve medical outcomes, even in facilities with exceedingly dire conditions.[28]

An Israeli study conducted at Hadassah-Hebrew University Medical Center hospitals in Jerusalem suggested that hand-hygiene compliance is influenced by "local culture." They were not referring to the heterogeneity of the population, rather to the culture and customs of medical practice in different hospital environments. The two hospitals studied, at the Ein Kerem and Mount Scopus campuses, differed in hand-hygiene compliance. (Mean adherence was 77 percent at Mount Scopus and 33 percent at Ein Kerem.) But they also differed in quality of facilities, as the older hospital at Ein Kerem had fewer sinks in patient rooms, for instance. In addition, attitudes among staff differed, with Cantrell and coworkers suggesting that Ein Kerem staff believed they worked harder, since that branch got more complex cases.[29]

In addition to differences between the two hospitals, there appeared to be differences in the culture between medical disciplines and specialties, leading to dramatic differences in handwashing compliance from ward to ward. For instance, some medical wards had very high compliance; that is, 91 percent in pediatrics and 96 percent in neonatal wards. Others had shockingly low compliance (14 percent in surgery as well as in the obstetrics wards). The authors suggest that pediatrics and neonatal intensive care units do better with regard to hand hygiene, because very young patients are seen as more vulnerable to complications from infections.[30]

While 96 percent compliance sounds impressive (a grade of A in most courses), the authors point out that despite such high compliance marks in neonatal ICUs, this was still unacceptable, since a baby who is touched ten times per day would have "more than 90 percent chance of exposure to at least one unclean hand in less than a week." They make the point that "effective prevention of nosocomial transmission requires an adherence rate of 100 percent."[31]

The same study concluded that making washing stations more available, and introducing and educating workers about alcohol-based hand rubs and the importance of compliance, were effective in raising compliance significantly and reducing risks in all wards of the hospitals.[32] However much those remedies help, it is possible to do more to improve hygiene.

Remedies
Changing Attitudes, Culture, and Thinking Styles

In the University of Toledo Medical Center study cited previously, it was found that educational level was inversely related to handwashing practice, with higher degrees of medical training associated with lower compliance. In a total of 2,373 observations, nurses demonstrated a very respectable 91.3 percent rate of handwashing compliance, but attending physicians had the lowest observed rate, 72.4 percent.[33] In the same hospital, after a visit by the Joint Commission on Accreditation of Healthcare Organizations (JCAHO), nurses further improved their hand-hygiene practices, perhaps in response to being assessed by members of the commission, but doctors did not.[34] Remediation appears to change behavior for some individuals under some circumstances, but not for everyone. Traditional and novel approaches to modifying hand-hygiene behavior will be addressed in depth in chapter 5.

People also tend to behave differently at different times of the day. In the Duggan et al. study, handwashing compliance was significantly higher from Monday through Wednesday, compared with Thursday and Friday, and it was significantly better from 3 P.M. through 11 P.M. compared to 7 A.M. to 3 P.M.[35] Motivation and energy levels tend to ebb and flow during the day, which might explain differences in compliance between the morning and evening shifts. I would have thought that handwashing behavior would be better during the day shift rather than the evening shift, but the opposite was reported, possibly because that shift tends to be less hectic and there is more time to wash. People also tend to feel and act differently at the end of the week, perhaps showing symptoms of TGIF ("Thank God It's Friday") syndrome.

Can we change behavior to improve the handwashing compliance of doctors who may feel that they do not need direction? Can we overcome the issues of authority and status and get the people at the top of the medical totem pole to comply? Can we address the issue of fluctuations in energy and motivation in the daily and weekly cycles? These issues may not be easy to tackle, but there are creative strategies we can use to improve hand hygiene.

CHANGE THINKING STYLES

Thinking styles may influence hand hygiene in clinical settings. An Australian study looked at the relationship between rational thinking and experiential thinking as they apply to hand-hygiene compliance.[36] Rational thinking refers to analytical, logical, and conscious processes; learning a new skill, as with driving a car, involves rational, active, focused, and conscious processes. Experiential thinking is more passive and automatic; it is mediated by practice and experience, and is the type of thinking used for habitual behaviors. For instance, the act of driving as an experienced driver involves experiential thinking. "Compliance was significantly positively correlated with experiential/automatic thinking." The study concluded that "hand hygiene is more experiential than rational . . . traditional approaches based on logic and reasoning alone probably will not work."[37] Any behavior that becomes habitual is more likely to be repeated and become a routine action. This includes harmful behaviors, such as smoking; neutral behaviors, such as driving a car; and beneficial behaviors, such as brushing teeth. The Weight Watchers program includes a food plan and recommendations for exercise and activity, but most important, it includes behavioral modifications and approaches to change attitudes and actions related to eating. Those who are most successful in the program develop new habits that become "routines," "feel second nature,"[38] and become automatic, guided by experiential thinking. If we can transform good hand-hygiene behaviors into habitual, automatic acts guided by experiential thinking, there is a better chance that medical personnel, and indeed, all of us, will practice it.

CHANGE THE CULTURE

Research at Hadassah Medical Center in Jerusalem showed a difference in "culture" between two hospitals, and between various wards.[39] The behavior of personnel appears to differ based on training, administrative attitudes, norms of the medical disciplines, and other factors that are hard to define.

In order to effectively change behavior, it is necessary to change culture, beliefs, and priorities. First, it is important to demonstrate the benefits of handwashing. In many cases, computation of a cost/benefit ratio may be convincing. If the cost in time, effort, and money is high, then the benefit must likewise be high to make the behavior worthwhile. If a doctor considers an action, such as handwashing, as time consuming or inconvenient, then the benefits of that action must be clearly spelled out in terms of improved health, reduced complications, and better patient outcomes. In addition, the risks of noncompliance must be obvious: increased medical complications caused by infection, reduced health and quality of life of patients, increased risk of higher mortality rates, and exposure to malpractice claims.

Researchers from Brisbane and Sydney, Australia, addressed the issue of how to change handwashing behavior. When nurses were provided with alcoholic hand rubs, intended to make it more convenient to wash, it led to a small increase in handwashing. But the factors that influenced handwashing in nurses most strongly were the nurses' belief in the benefits of the action, peer pressure from senior physicians and administrators, and role modeling. Doctors can also be swayed by convincing evidence, including sharing the results of research studies, and cost/benefit analysis with regard to outcomes. The authors conclude that the "introduction of hand rub alone without an associated behavioral modification program is unlikely to induce a sustained increase in hand hygiene compliance."[40]

TELL THE TRUTH

It is critical when studying the issue of hand hygiene in healthcare facilities to make sure that the research approach actually measures what is happening. Some studies involve self-reporting by medical personnel of their own behavior, while others use direct observation of behavior by outside observers. Which approach is more accurate? If there is a motive to stretch the truth or even lie, will this influence self-reporting? A British study compared self-reporting of handwashing practices by healthcare workers to observed behaviors. The authors found a "discrepancy between self-reported and observed hand hygiene behaviour in healthcare professionals."[41] The research followed seventy-one healthcare workers, comparing self-reporting on questionnaires about handwashing with the observation of actual behavior.

In that study the authors defined "opportunity for hand hygiene" as "any occasion when a participant performed any activity that required hand hygiene, including contact with the patient, equipment, medication or food, or prior to carers going on their break."[42] Using that definition, they observed 1,284 hand-hygiene opportunities over the course of 132 hours.

The authors of the study broadly defined hand hygiene as "any attempt to clean hands with water alone, with water and one of the available handwashing products, or with alcohol-based hand rub."[43] The method used and the duration of the action were not measured or judged.

First, the data reveal that hand hygiene in their facility leaves something to be desired. The data collected by direct observation revealed that hand-washing practices were poor, even though the caretakers were aware that they were being observed. For all contacts, in 642 observed opportunities, only 12 percent of caretakers washed their hands both before and after the activity. An additional 20 percent only washed before and 61 percent only washed after the activity. Seven percent of the time the caretaker did not wash at all.

This is of concern since the activities included contact with patients— moving; examining; feeding; administration of medications by mouth, by nasogastric tube, and intravenously; catheterization; and even contact with MRSA. For instance, in wound management (seven observations), only one person washed hands both before and after the activity; five people washed only after touching the patient; and one person did not wash at all, either before or after contact. In fifty contacts with MRSA patients, 16 percent washed before and after, 6 percent washed only before, 62 percent washed only after the activity and 16 percent did not wash their hands at all.

Further analysis of the data shows that in activities judged to be high risk for infection of the patient, 19 percent washed before and after, and an additional 26 percent washed only before the activity. This means that for most of the contacts (55 percent) where infection of the patient was a high risk, no washing took place before the activity. However, when the risk of infection to the caretaker was high, 13 percent washed before and after, and an additional 81 percent washed only after contact, totaling 94 percent of caretakers who washed after contact when there was high risk to themselves.

In the same study, when behavior of specific occupational groups are analyzed, healthcare assistants came out the best with 23.3 percent washing hands before an activity and 65 percent after. Qualified nurses were the second-best hand washers (20.4 percent before, 60.1 percent after), and doctors and therapists both lagged far behind (doctors washed 8.1 percent of the time before the activity and 51.4 percent after; therapists washed 6.3 percent of the time before and 87.5 percent of the time after the activity). None of these statistics inspire confidence in the medical personnel in this institution. Clearly these numbers of observed behaviors are very far from perfect. But the story only gets worse. The healthcare workers, including highly trained doctors and nurses, either think they are doing better, or just lie outright about their handwashing records.

The questionnaires in which medical personnel self-reported on their hand-hygiene behavior were analyzed and compared to observed behaviors. Questions included a section to reveal the attitudes and intentions of caretakers as well as their self-reporting of behaviors. The authors found a significant relationship between attitudes on hand hygiene and intention to perform hand hygiene. In other words, if they believed it was valuable, they expressed the intention to do it. However, "self-reported hand hygiene behaviour was not related at all to actual observations."[44] That is to say, many of the healthcare personnel did not, after all, execute their intentions. It is not clear why this discrepancy exists. It could be a matter of misreporting, overestimating, covering up, or fabrication. Perhaps there is pressure to perform and overreporting is a way to save face.

The authors conclude that interventions meant to change attitudes and intentions will not necessarily ensure action. The study revealed a disconnect between what people say they believe in and intend to do, and their actual behavior. Even if someone is convinced that it is a good thing to wash hands, it does not necessarily translate into handwashing. In this study, the data suggested "that hand hygiene interventions that target changes in attitudes, intentions or self-reported practice are likely to fail in terms of changing behavior."[45]

Given the conclusions of Jenner et al. that "healthcare professionals clean their hands much less often than they say they do,"[46] what can be done to improve the situation? Even when they knew they were being watched, the actual handwashing record was far from perfect. Clearly more education, clarification of expectations, and changing of practices is needed. But better follow-up is also critical to ensure that the intentions are translated into actions. Furthermore, any assessment of handwashing in medical settings must be done by direct observation of behavior and not by self-reporting, since the medical personnel in this study may have overestimated, exaggerated, or fabricated their reports.

The authors of the study recommend a program they developed called Dynamic Assessment Strategy for Hand Hygiene (DASHH). It involves teaching caretakers to "consider hand hygiene before and after care as separate activities requiring separate risk assessments."[47] Before every activity, the caretaker must determine the level of risk to the patient with regard to infection. After every activity, the caretaker must determine the level of risk to self and to other patients. Based on the two separate assessments, appropriate hand-hygiene strategy must be employed both before interacting with a patient and after the event. And this must be done every time patient care is initiated, without exceptions. "Such a strategy provides healthcare professionals with a simple mental map to make the quick informed decisions that are required when busy on a ward," conclude the authors.[48]

While this approach appears rational and its intentions are noble, the proposed method needs to be validated as an effective strategy. Best practices for measuring compliance have proven to be elusive, as attested to by American researchers who attempted to measure and compare hand hygiene across healthcare organizations. The goal of that study was "to identify promising and effective practices for measuring adherence with hand hygiene guidelines across a variety of settings."[49] They collected data on 242 healthcare organizations and facilities, from different countries, reporting vast inconsistencies in the types of hand-hygiene data collected. Only 75 percent of respondents measured the frequency of hand hygiene, and about half of the sample measured other factors, such as thoroughness of washing, use of gloves, and use of cleansers. The study revealed that there is little standardization worldwide in how hand hygiene compliance is monitored and reported, and there is "little evidence of reliability."[50]

Disclosure of Infection of Medical Personnel

Another disturbing issue is the prospect of risk posed by an infected healthcare worker who has a serious infectious disease. "When the Surgeon Is Infected, How Safe Is the Surgery?" asks the author of a *New York Times* article.[51] It tells the story of two Long Island residents who, while attending a support group for individuals infected with Hepatitis C, discover by chance that they shared the same surgeon. Further medical inquiry revealed that the surgeon, Dr. Michael Hall, was infected with the Hepatitis C virus and had transmitted it unknowingly to both patients. Janine

Jagger, an epidemiologist who has studied clinical safety and reduction of risk to medical personnel, explains that the transmission of infections from patients to medical workers has been studied and documented for centuries. The reverse problem, transmission from medical personnel to patients, while much less common, can and also does occur. "Patients never suspect this could happen to them," said Jagger. "It's really swept under the carpet."[52]

In "Unwashed Doctors," Dr. Thomas Papadimos declares his frustration that "grown men and women who call themselves 'Doctor' cannot even take the time to wash their hands . . . [T]his is a travesty in regard to patient safety. I do not care how many papers you have published, or how many patients or dollars you draw to the hospital, you are on notice, sir or madam, that your behavior is no longer to be tolerated. Fines and suspension may face you in the days ahead."[53] In his Letter to the Editor of a prestigious scientific journal, Papadimos continues his unorthodox rant, "What kind of arrogance prevents us from washing our hands when we enter a patient's room, and what halts colleagues and other health workers from pointing it out to the offenders? I have no good answer. Hand washing is one of the bedrocks of patient safety."[54]

Dr. Guy Maddern takes the outrage further, "The cavalier attitude of some surgeons and surgical trainees to the most basic steps associated with good hand washing in the wards, let alone the operating theatre never ceases to amaze. . . . When simple measures such as hand washing between patients and better infection control behaviour in theatres can have such a lasting impact the noncompliant individual surgeon or trainee should be moved to non-clinical duties or early retirement."[55]

Proper patient care has more issues to consider than the simple act of handwashing, but clearly hand hygiene is of major concern. The hygiene situation in medical settings seems rather hopeless, yet there is hope and there are strategies we can implement, short of firing the unwashed, to reduce risk and stay healthy. "Ask Me If I Washed My Hands" is one campaign that has many supporters. An editorial by medical writer Suzanne Gordon, which appeared in the prestigious medical journal _JAMA_ (_The Journal of the American Medical Association_), discusses such initiatives. Gordon reported an anecdote about a medical intern and a medical resident who observed their attending physician examine three patients in a row, without washing his hands. Despite the fact that one of those patients had MRSA, neither junior doctor said a word to the attending about his omission. Gordon recounted her own experience as a patient treated by a nurse who failed to wash her hands—the author also failed to ask the nurse to wash her hands, even though her own health was at risk. She felt she would be at greater risk if she confronted the nurse and made her angry. "This woman had the power to hurt me and I was afraid to anger her."[56] Gordon reports that it is quite common for patients, who are vulnerable and dependent, to be unable to assert themselves on this issue. One remedy she suggests is to establish a culture and environment where physicians and nurses convincingly and decisively "order" their patients to remind them to clean their hands. Her second proposal is to establish a code word that colleagues or patients could use to flag the violation before the medical practitioner touches a patient. "But the only way this will work is if hospital and health care administrators make it crystal clear that they will back up anyone who challenges a person senior to themselves to enforce hand hygiene and that expressing such concern is not only an acceptable but expected action."[57] The magic word suggested by Gordon is "Hands!"[58]

I have, on occasion, used a similar strategy when faced with food handlers manhandling my pizza. I politely ask them to serve me the slice without using hands. Of course, in that situation I am not a vulnerable patient lying on a gurney in a hospital gown. I am a paying customer. I am empowered.

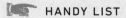 HANDY LIST

*How to Reduce Your Risk of Infection as
a Patient in a Healthcare Facility*

1 Keep yourself clean; wash your own hands regularly, especially after
   using the bathroom and before eating. This might not be as easy as
   it sounds, especially if you are bedridden or have difficulty getting
   to a sink. You will need to be assertive and ask for assistance with
   handwashing and hygiene.

2 Remind and insist that anyone who is going to touch you, for medical
   or personal reasons, wash their hands. This includes your visitors,
   family, and loved ones, who most likely just came in off the street and
   are carrying microbes from the outside environment. Remind them
   to wash their hands again before they leave the facility, to protect
   themselves from carrying home germs.

3 Be aware, to the best of your ability, of any medical devices,
   instruments, or surfaces you encounter. Are they packaged, sterile,
   and new? If not, have they been disinfected just before use? Are
   surfaces such as exam tables covered so your skin does not touch
   them? Was the linen being used taken from a freshly laundered pile?
   If you are too ill to monitor this, ask a trusted friend or family member
   to be your advocate for hygiene, in addition to monitoring your medical
   treatment.

4 This is so important that it warrants repeating: ask all medical
   personnel to wash their hands before touching you. And if they touch
   any of your body parts that might be particularly germ-laden (genitals,
   anus, skin sores, soiled bedding, urinary catheter and bag), they
   should wash again before tending to your wounds, IV lines, PICC lines
   (peripherally inserted central catheter), or your eyes, nose, mouth, or
   throat (tracheotomy).

5 Ask medical personnel to wear gloves and to change them when
   warranted. If the doctor or nurse touches germ-laden surfaces, they
   should change their gloves before touching you. Insist on this, or ask
   your advocate to make this point in a polite and respectful way.

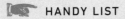 **HANDY LIST**

When Should Healthcare Workers Perform Hand Hygiene?

1 Before patient contact
2 After contact with patient's skin
3 After contact with patient's gown or linen
4 After contact with inanimate objects in patient's room
5 Before and after IV care
6 Before and after IV insertion
7 Before and after wound contact
8 Before and after mucous membrane contact
9 Before and after body fluid contact

Source: John M. Boyce and Didier Pittet, "Guideline for Hand Hygiene in Health-Care Settings: Recommendations of the Healthcare Infection Control Practices Advisory Committee and the HICPAC/SHEA/APIC/IDSA Hand Hygiene Task Force," *American Journal of Infection Control* 30 (2002): S1–S46.

Touch at Your Own Risk

Philadelphia's Please Touch Museum is a delightful facility where small children can enjoy a variety of experiences, with exhibits designed for the very youngest explorers. As anyone who has had a toddler knows, children love to, in fact, they *have* to touch everything. Touching is one of the major ways that children learn about the world. So a museum that encourages touching is on the right wavelength for tots. At the Please Touch Museum there is a pretend supermarket, make-believe trucks, a SEPTA bus (SEPTA is Philadelphia's subway system), a hospital featuring a miniature CT scan for dolls, an imagination playground, a carousel, and water play exhibits. All of these exhibits are designed to be touched by children under the age of seven, over and over again, producing an environment conducive to the transfer of microbes from child to surfaces to child. This is not a new phenomenon, as touching and transferring germs happens in every school, day care, or playground frequented by small children. Even the waiting room in a pediatrician's office can be a vector of transmission of germs—and a place to get sick. My children's pediatrician did his best to minimize contagious children passing on microbes to healthy ones by providing two waiting areas, one for sick children and one for healthy children. He has an appreciation for the problem of contaminated surfaces being a source of infection. But touching and sharing germs is sure to happen, regardless of precautions, wherever small children congregate.

Girolamo Fracastoro, who lived some five hundred years ago (introduced in chapter 2) and was the first to propose germs as agents of infectious disease, also recognized that surfaces can be contaminated and transmit disease. He coined the term "fome," for germ-laden surfaces, when he wrote, "There are, it seems, three fundamentally different types of contagion: the first infects by direct contact only, the second does the same, but in addition leaves fomes, and this contagion may spread by means of that fomes . . . By fomes I mean clothes, wooden objects, and things of that sort, which though not themselves corrupted can, nevertheless, preserve the original germs of the contagion and infect by means of these; thirdly, there is a kind of contagion which is transmitted not only by direct contact or by fomes as intermediary, but also infects at a distance."[1] *Fomes* is the Latin word for tinder, material that readily ignites to help one start a fire. The seeds of contagion were understood to be able to spread just as the flickering of a flaming tinder can spread to other materials. Today we use the term *fomite* to refer to an object or surface that carries germs and can transmit them from one person to another.

With great insight, Fracastoro observed that germs can reside and survive on surfaces for long periods of time. He wrote, "The principle that exists in fomes seems to be of a different nature, inasmuch as, when it has retired into fomes from the body originally infected, it may last there for a very long time without any alteration. Things that have been touched by persons suffering from phthisis or the plague are really amazing examples of this. I have often observed that in them this virus has been preserved for two or three years."[2]

Fracastoro was right on target. Things that are touched by sick people can become contaminated, and the germs, that is, bacteria or viruses, can survive on surfaces for long periods of time. It is important to be aware of the risks posed by different environmental surfaces and what types of precautions we can take to minimize exposure to harmful microbes. Even the most meticulous hand washer is at risk of picking up infectious agents from the environment. In chapter 1 we discussed microbiomes: home microbiomes, office microbiomes, and even the New York City Subway microbiome, where 1,688 different microbes were found. If you touch environmental surfaces, regardless of where you are on our living planet, you will pick up microorganisms. For the most part the microbes are benign, but there is always a risk of transferring pathogenic germs from a contaminated surface to your own hands, and then to your mouth or other part of your body, where the microbes could make you ill.

Fomites that pose the highest risks are things that we touch the most with our hands: doorknobs, toilet and sink handles, our clothes and other fabrics around us, coins and paper money, rings, handbags, cell phones, and even latex gloves that we might wear to protect us and others from the transfer of germs. In clinical settings those very same gloves, as well as instruments and other devices used in patient care, can be carriers of disease.

An episode of the popular TV show *Scrubs*[3] dramatized the transfer of deadly germs from one person to another. Throughout the episode an infectious agent appears in the hospital as a bright green stain wherever it is: on people's hands, a glove, a trash can. At the end of the episode an incompetent intern picks up a contaminated glove from the hospital floor and throws it away. He then shakes hands with a beloved elderly patient, transferring the germs, a green stain of death, to her. This episode dramatically illustrates how dangerous contaminated objects can be and how we need to be aware of the risks of transmitting disease by touching objects and each other's hands.

The "Five-Second Rule"

This brings us to one of the most common hygiene issues people encounter: If food falls on the floor, is it wise to eat it or does it pose a risk? Those who invoke the "Five-Second Rule" believe that if the food is recovered within five seconds of dropping it, then it is still safe to eat. However, that is not a reliable rule because, depending on the type of food and where it is dropped, food can pick up germs immediately. Connecticut College students compared apple slices and Skittles candy that were left on the college dining-hall floor for various intervals. Moist or wet food is much more likely to become contaminated quickly, and the apple slices picked up germs much faster than the Skittles. But location is also an essential issue. If your candy falls on a hot sidewalk that has been baking in the summer sun, that surface may be almost germfree because, as Supreme Court Justice Louis Brandeis noted, "Sunlight is said to be the best of disinfectants."[4] (His quote was referring to transparency in disclosing information for public scrutiny, but it also applies to germs and sunbaked surfaces.) A sidewalk that has been baking in the sun for hours may be a low-risk zone, and food dropped on such a surface may remain relatively germfree. However, moist soil alongside that sidewalk, can harbor a broad spectrum of living organisms, including microbes that pose a danger to human health. Bathroom and kitchen floors can be particularly high-risk zones, as bathrooms may harbor bacteria and viruses from human waste and kitchens may have more germs from contaminated foods. Those floors may be contaminated with microbes such as *E. coli* and *Salmonella*, therefore the bathroom and kitchen floors should be considered "zero-second zones."[5] So if your food falls on the floor, it is important to ask—what food and which floor?

Clothing and Other Textiles or Fabrics

I once observed a tie-wearing physician bend over a young patient, his tie sweeping across the child's abdomen. I imagined how many tummies that tie had touched and where else that tie had been, and I became concerned that the tie could carry germs from doctor to patient or from one patient to the tie to another patient. Most doctors will typically see a number of patients in a short span of time, going directly from patient to patient. Could a necktie harbor microbes long enough to carry infections and transfer germs from one person to another? Two British studies found evidence to support this likelihood.

In the orthopedic department of a Surrey hospital, they discovered that doctors' ties carry pathogenic microbes that matched the germs from their patients' infected wounds. "We lean towards our patients on a regular basis while examining them, either the tie is hanging freely and able to touch the patient or is tucked into the shirt and bacteria are transferred indirectly by the hands," noted the authors.[6] Based on a number of such observations, the British Medical Association recommended in 2006 that doctors not wear neckties on clinical rounds, as they may put patients at risk of infection.[7]

Despite these recommendations, three years later in a London hospital researchers tested the neckties and shirts of fifty doctors for the presence of bacterial contamination. As might be expected, all of the doctors reported that they had worn their shirts for fewer than two days since they were last laundered. With regard to neckties, however, "Sixteen had never cleaned their tie, and 20 could not remember when they had cleaned it. For the remaining 14, the mean time since the last cleaning of their tie was 73 days." There were significantly higher bacterial counts on ties compared with shirts, suggesting that washable clothing is preferable in clinical settings.[8]

In my laboratory at William Paterson University, we study the interaction of bacteria with different types of fabrics and other surfaces. Our studies on polyester and silk from neckties demonstrated that most ties harbor living bacteria for long periods of time. There are many opportunities for fabrics to pick up germs. Natural fibers and fabrics can become contaminated during growth (wools come from animal fleeces, silk comes from silkworm cocoons, and cotton and linen are from plants). Natural or artificial fibers can acquire microbes during the preparation or synthesis of fibers (from natural or synthetic sources); during handling in the dyeing, weaving, or knitting processes; in sale, shipment, or stocking; and by consumer handling. Contaminating bacteria or other microbes can survive on the fabrics for long periods of time and can be transferred from fabrics to other surfaces and back again.

In our experiments we prepared swatches from numerous samples of ties (used ties and newly purchased ones) and placed them in petri dishes on nutrient agar to encourage the reproduction of bacteria found on the fabrics. Some samples were free of growth, but in many samples dormant or residual bacteria emerged from the fibers and flourished in the culture dishes. On silk samples we observed a film of bacteria and clusters of bacterial colonies across the surface as well as around the edges of the fabric. Polyester samples showed bacterial growth around the edges with little growth on the surface. There are incidental bacteria and other microbes on fabrics that have been handled by people through the manufacturing, transport, and sale of the material. Since we do not live in a sterile world, microbes are ubiquitous. The bacteria we found appeared to be common strains found in the everyday environment. A major question that needed to be addressed was whether fabrics can be deliberately contaminated with other bacterial species, and if so, will new bacteria compete with resident flora and crowd them out?[9] This was meant to simulate what can happen in a healthcare environment when disease-associated bacteria hitch a ride on clothing and endanger patients.

We developed a method to contaminate different fabrics with various strains of bacteria, and tested them again. When we exposed the swatches to *E. coli*, they readily picked up the microbes, and the *E. coli* became a dominant species on the surface of many samples, outgrowing the resident bacteria. Similar results were obtained with *Staphylococcus epider-*

midis and *Bacillus subtilis*.[10] The three strains of bacteria we used in these experiments do not pose serious health risks in the laboratory, but they were chosen to simulate what happens with disease-causing bacteria. We used three strains that have different cell characteristics (*Escherichia coli* are gram negative rods, *Bacillus subtilis* are gram positive rods, and *Staphylococcus epidermidis* are gram positive cocci) to simulate a variety of pathogens. Based on these results, we believe it is likely that fabrics can pick up disease-causing pathogenic species, when touched by germ-carrying individuals.

Given that fabrics can acquire microbes, the next step was to study methods to destroy or remove the contaminants. Soaps and detergents primarily work by mechanically removing microbes from surfaces, such as fabrics and skin. Some soaps and detergents also disrupt the integrity of bacterial cells as well as viruses. Thus, laundering with detergent should reduce or eliminate germs, and it is a good way to disinfect contaminated clothes, bedding, and other materials. But not every garment is wash and wear; neither is it always convenient to launder cloth between uses. As we learned from the British tie study (and you probably know from your own experience), people rarely or never clean their ties, as tie fabrics do not fare well in the laundry. So how can we keep ties from becoming disease vectors?

We tested a variety of approaches to disinfect fabrics, with mixed results. For instance, we found that treatment with the antibiotics penicillin and streptomycin reduced or eliminated bacteria on silk, but not from polyester. Of course, using antibiotics to disinfect ties or other textiles would not be very practical, as antibiotics are expensive and would needlessly expose humans to those drugs. Treatment of swatches with 70 percent ethyl alcohol reduced or eliminated bacterial growth from polyester but not from silk. Alcohol treatment is also not useful, as it caused bleeding of dyes from some of the tie fabrics.[11]

We expanded the project to study the three laboratory strains of bacteria, *E. coli*, *B. subtilis*, and *S. epidermidis*, on six different fabrics: polyester, silk, cotton, and wool (all from neckties); a polyester/cotton blend (from medical scrubs); and a microfiber fabric (from stain-resistant tablecloths). After contaminating the fabrics with bacteria, we tested various methods for disinfection: dry heat, steam heat, dry-cleaning fluid, heat lamp, ultraviolet radiation, and microwave treatment.[12]

Swatches exposed to *E. coli* and then heated with a dry iron showed mixed results; some samples had bacterial growth, and others appeared to be bacteria-free. Steam ironing was more effective and reduced, but did not eliminate, *E. coli* in most samples. We exposed swatches of contaminated material to dry cleaning fluid, expecting that such noxious chemicals would be highly effective in decontaminating the fabrics. Surprisingly, in most cases dry cleaning fluid did not kill the bacteria. In fact, in some samples dry cleaning fluid appeared to enhance or support bacterial growth. This is consistent with the ability of some bacteria to use the chemicals as food—they can metabolize organic chemicals (a process called biodegradation), however noxious they may be. We learned that many dry cleaning establishments add antibacterial chemicals to the dry cleaning solutions in order to prevent the growth of bacteria in those fluids.[13]

We tried to disinfect contaminated swatches (six different materials) with a heat lamp or uv radiation, both methods that are said to kill germs, but it did not reduce bacterial contamination. Although "sunlight is . . . the best disinfectant" (which is marginally true—it can reduce the population of microbes, but does not sterilize surfaces), perhaps the heat lamp was not hot enough or used long enough to have an effect. It is possible that ultraviolet radiation did not work because the radiation cannot penetrate past the top surface and into deeper fibers. Even microwaving the swatches for two minutes in a conventional microwave oven was ineffective in killing all the bacteria.[14] Clearly, it is not as easy to disinfect cloth as we thought it would be.

One important question was how long can microbes linger on surfaces, alive and still able to infect? The longer the germs linger, the higher the risk that they will be transmitted from one surface to another or to another person. In one hospital study staphylococci and enterococci survived more than ninety days on fabrics and plastic in clinical settings.[15] We conducted experiments to determine if bacteria-contaminated surfaces typically found in clinics, hospitals, homes, and schools (namely, glass, paper, plastic, and four different fabrics) can transfer living cells to other surfaces. One day after exposure to bacteria, living bacteria were transferred from surface to surface. Bacteria were transferred from glass, paper, and plastic to scrubs, nylon, silk, and microfiber. Likewise, bacteria on scrubs, nylon, silk, and microfiber transferred to glass, paper, or plastic. Additional experiments showed that bacteria readily transfer between wood and glass surfaces, and between wood and stainless steel, other surfaces commonly found in our environments.

In one experiment we treated seven surfaces (scrubs, microfiber, nylon, silk, glass, paper, and plastic) with *B. subtilis* and waited five days. After five days viable bacteria still transferred from surface to surface. We noted a few exceptions: *B. subtilis* on microfiber did not transfer to plastic, paper, or glass. In addition, there was no transfer from plastic to nylon, or from silk to glass. We would be interested in learning more about plastic/nylon and silk/glass interactions. But more remarkably, in numerous experiments, microfiber appeared to be different from other fabrics. Microfiber is a synthetic material made of very finespun artificial threads. The type we used came from stain-repellent tablecloths and is very hydrophobic; in other words, it repels water. We observed that samples of microfiber were different from the other fabrics in that bacteria grew to a lesser extent, or not at all, on microfiber. In addition, when we looked at individual bacteria-treated microfiber threads in the microscope, the threads were clean and bacteria-free, compared with other textiles that were teeming with microbes. It appears that microfiber is able to repel bacteria, possibly because it repels water or any watery environment in which bacteria are suspended.[16] Perhaps microfiber would be a good fabric to use in clinical settings, as it is less likely to retain or transfer bacteria to other surfaces. It might be used in clothing that is at high risk of contamination, such as sleeves, cuffs, and the front of shirts.

After numerous experiments we discovered that the best antibacterial treatment for all the fabrics we tested was 3 percent hydrogen peroxide. Hydrogen peroxide is a cheap and readily available liquid that is sold in pharmacies in brown glass or plastic bottles. The three bacterial strains were highly sensitive to hydrogen peroxide regardless of which fabric was used. *E. coli* and *B. subtilis* were completely eliminated, while *S. epidermidis* was reduced by more than 90 percent. While hydrogen peroxide is sometimes used to bleach hair, the fabrics we tested did not appear to be damaged by exposure to 3 percent hydrogen peroxide—there was no fading, leeching of dye, or changing of color. However, we only tested small swatches, not intact ties, so the question of how damaging hydrogen peroxide would be to sensitive materials is still open, and the practical applicability of hydrogen peroxide as a tie disinfectant remains unsettled.

What we do know is that necktie fabrics can harbor bacteria for days, weeks, or months; and neckties are worn by some men day in and day out, and are rarely washed or dry cleaned by their owners. Can neckties harbor and transfer microbes? Indeed, they do, and since men rarely wash or dry clean their ties, any contaminant that hops aboard the tie material can be carried all day, day after day, wherever the man roams.

Latex Gloves

One recommended approach to avoid germs that has become policy in many healthcare settings as well as for food preparation is the wearing of disposable latex gloves. Wearing gloves helps to protect the person wearing the gloves from picking up potentially harmful germs. It also protects others from direct contact with the hands of the wearer. Latex gloves became a consistent part of healthcare policy during the AIDS epidemic of the 1980s. In light of a new infectious disease for which there was no cure, healthcare workers would no longer take their chances on being exposed to blood or other bodily fluids, so gloving became routine and recommended. Latex and other types of disposable gloves serve as a protective barrier to reduce the risk of transmission of germs from person to person, but they only work well if they are used properly. If the person wearing gloves contaminates the gloves by touching a germ-laden surface, the gloves themselves can become a vector of disease and can spread the germs more widely, as there is a false sense of security when your hands are covered in latex. The California Child Care Health Program curriculum for training child-care workers instructs that workers should never wear gloves *instead of* washing hands. Hands must always be washed before and after certain tasks, regardless of whether gloves are worn. While gloves do serve as a barrier and can protect the worker from contamination, gloves are easily breached. Handwashing is still the primary approach to reducing the risk of spreading germs.[17]

"Best practices" dictate that gloves should be changed regularly if they become contaminated or breached. One issue that may not be so obvious, even in a hospital environment, is that the glove box itself can become hazardous. At the "First Hospital Microbiome Project" workshop scientists discussed that issue, noting that when a person reaches into the box of disposable gloves, the fingers come into contact with many gloves, contaminating their surfaces. The next person to take gloves out of the box may be exposed to any microbes left behind by that other individual. Thus, they noted that glove use has problems, and handwashing remains "the single most effective measure in preventing hospital-acquired infections."[18]

In child-care settings, the recommendations are to wear gloves when contact with blood is likely, for instance, if a child's cut is being cleansed or bandaged, or if the caregiver herself has open cuts or sores on her hand. In addition, gloves should be worn when cleaning or handling clothing or other items that are soiled with bodily wastes, or when caring for a child requires the touching of mouth or eyes. Many child-care facilities require gloves for diaper changes; if they are used, they should be changed between diaper changes from one child to another. Regardless of the glove usage policy, hands always should be washed between diaper changes. It is a good idea to keep gloves handy, at the diaper-changing table, in the playground, and with the first-aid supplies in case issues arise that will expose workers to blood or other bodily fluids.[19]

Healthcare workers are trained and become aware of procedures involving gloves. Gloves are used in the workplace where chemicals and other hazardous materials are used, and where food preparation is done, to protect the product as well as the worker. One article regarding the use of gloves by factory workers states "best practice" regarding their use: "Gloves must be in good condition to protect the hands . . . to keep materials from penetrating the skin. They should fit properly . . . be kept clean, and be discarded when they become worn out or grossly contaminated . . . [W]earing gloves without practicing good hygiene is no more protective than not wearing gloves at all."[20] Although this appears to be an obvious commonsense approach to glove use, it needs to be explicitly stated, or workers may be unaware that tattered gloves—or even a glove with one hole—have little to no protective value.

When considering food safety, New York City food carts do not spring to mind as the safest places to eat. The incidence of food-borne diseases that occur because of the transmission of pathogens by food workers is of great concern since one in six Americans reportedly suffer from food-borne diseases every year.[21] The New York City Health Code requires that food workers change their gloves after handling money or before they touch food. However, a study of food vendor carts in New York City showed that almost 57 percent of the time food vendors did not change their gloves after touching money.[22] This is not surprising since food carts do not have much supervision, the food handlers do not have training in this area, and transactions can occur in rapid succession, with little time to change gloves. Even if they have the time, the food handlers may not wish to change gloves, as this can become a very expensive practice.

Since many vendors are using the same gloves to handle money and food, we wanted to determine if money handled by those vendors was con-taminated with bacteria. Twenty-five New York City food vendors situated near various hospitals were observed for one hour each. In the course of 495 monetary transactions observed, there were only seven glove changes performed by the workers. At the end of each one-hour observation period, we conducted a transaction with each vendor, in which we received a dollar bill as change. (To prevent any further contamination, the observers used sterile gloves to receive the dollar bill, and they placed the bill directly into sterile tryptic soy broth in a sterile tube.) Nineteen out of twenty-five dollar bills we received as change from the twenty-five vendors were contami-nated with bacteria, and ten of those tested positive for coliform bacteria.[23]

In our "pizza parlor" experiment, we simulated what might happen in a pizza shop or other food establishment when a worker fails to change gloves after handling money. We exposed samples of paper currency (cut from one-dollar bills) to *E. coli*, *B. subtilis*, or *S. epidermidis* and allowed the "dirty money" to sit at room temperature for various periods of time, up to several days. The "dirty money" samples were then briefly applied to samples cut from sterile latex gloves. The results showed that in all cases bacteria transferred from the paper currency to the latex gloves. In order to develop an approach to reduce the risk of dirty gloves transferring mi-crobes to food, we contaminated latex with bacteria, then treated it with alcohol-based hand sanitizer or with 3 percent hydrogen peroxide. Both methods worked to eliminate bacteria on the glove latex.[24] This suggests that if food handlers are reluctant to keep changing gloves because of the cost or inconvenience, they could at least quickly and conveniently sanitize their gloves with a squirt or two of hand sanitizer or hydrogen peroxide. This would reduce the risk of spreading contamination from surface to surface in food establishments.

It is not surprising that people who have no medical training may misuse gloves. The lack of awareness of how materials become contaminated and how microbes can be passed from one surface to another, as well as from one individual to another, leads to situations in which the gloves themselves are the problem, carrying germs from person to person. Medical personnel, who are trained in use of gloves, also need to be vigilant and to be mindful of gloves as a vector for the spread of disease. This sounds like common sense. However, if one is a regular glove user, it is easy to take the protection afforded by gloves for granted. Even if gloves are used conscientiously, there are potential problems if there is a breach in the glove. One study found perforations, on average, in 17 percent of surgeon's gloves.[25] Another study describes "invisible perforations" in as many as 82.5 percent of gloves and reports that most surgeons remain unaware of perforations.[26] (Is it possible that a breached or porous glove killed my mother by infecting her in the hospital?) These studies recommend using two pairs at once, or double gloving. Because disposable gloves are so easy to tear or breach, when we use radioactive materials in the lab we always double glove to protect ourselves, as a rupture or perforation could lead to radioactive contamination of the skin, which would be difficult to detect, hazardous to health, and difficult to remove.

Michael Barza reports on a novel type of glove treated with microspheres, that is, tiny chemical-filled compartments, that activate in the presence of light or moisture to become antimicrobial. This advance could reduce the risk of transmission of disease-causing pathogens in food handling or clinical settings.[27] Enhand-CR is another type of high-tech glove, which is treated with "MicroGard" that kills microorganisms on contact.[28] Of course, changing contaminated gloves on a regular basis can also accomplish the same goal—reducing the spread of disease.

Money May Be Hazardous to Your Health

One of our research projects described previously demonstrated that paper money can become contaminated with various bacteria, which can be readily transferred to glove latex samples. Thus, food handlers who handle money should be wary about transferring microbes from money to food. "Failure to adequately sanitize hands, or use food handling tools (tongs, spoons, utensils, or baker/serving papers) between handling money and serving food, could put patrons at risk."[29] This is particularly true since there are infectious intestinal diseases that can be contracted by contact with a low dose of the pathogen. The so-called "greasy spoon" type of diner that is not vigilant about hygiene in this manner could be a source of food-borne illness for many consumers.

How dirty is money? Is there a genuine risk involved from contaminated bills or coins? The U.S. Treasury prints about ten million one-dollar bills per day. Paper currency has an average life span of about eighteen months, and in that time the bills change hands numerous times. People use dollar bills in everyday exchanges on the street, in shops, in cafés, and as tips, and they shove those bills into wallets, purses, money clips, pockets, shoes, and G-strings. I have seen people who are already juggling a wallet, keys, and other personal items, grab a bill with their teeth before passing it on to pay for something. Some dollar bills fall into puddles, get dropped on the ground, are stepped on, or are washed and dried in the laundry. A purse full of my own coins and bills was submerged in the floodwaters of Superstorm Sandy. I salvaged that money and spread the coins and bills out to dry. Subsequently, some of that money was spent, and the rest was probably shoved into a drawer. In retrospect I wonder what was in that floodwater. There were likely many contaminants because of overflowing sewers and a mixing of seawater with dirty soil, mud, and other pollutants. At the time I did not give it much thought, but now that I am considering the situation, maybe that money should have been destroyed rather than passed on. I'd better go check my drawers for Sandy money and disinfect it properly. Or better yet, maybe I will use it for a research project.

Bills from many people and places get collected together in banks and cashier drawers and rub up against each other. So money gets around, and it gets exposed to many germs. As I mentioned earlier, my father, who loved to give money to his children and grandchildren, made a point of giving crisp, new bills from the bank. But most people don't care about the condition of their money; they are just concerned with how much they have.

It turns out that my dad was right about dirty money—it can carry germs that can make you sick. Our study of money from New York City food vendors discussed previously demonstrated that most of the dollar bills we received in change were contaminated.[30] Infectious disease researchers from Wright-Patterson Air Force Base in Ohio collected one-dollar bills from people in a checkout line at a local grocery store and at a concession stand in a high school basketball game. Anyone who had a dollar bill was eligible to participate, and everyone who was asked consented to be a participant. The volunteers were asked to roll up the bill and insert it into a tube of sterile nutrient broth. (They were then reimbursed with a new one-dollar bill.) The bills were soaked for thirty to sixty minutes in nutrient broth, and then removed from the liquid medium. The broth was incubated at 98.6 degrees F (human body temperature) to encourage any contaminating microbes to grow, then tested for the presence of bacteria. Five of the sixty-eight bills had pathogenic bacteria; another fifty-nine had potentially pathogenic strains, which could be dangerous to frail hospital or nursing home patients. That translates to 94 percent of the bills carrying bacteria of concern that could increase risk of infection.[31]

Money does get around from person to person and place to place. The website www.WheresGeorge.com follows U.S. currency as it moves from place to place around the country and outside the United States. The website, launched in 1998, enables people to monitor the movement of specific dollar bills as they are spent and move from person to person. Participants mark bills with "Where's George?" enter the serial number on the website, and then go spend the bill. They can check in periodically to see if anyone has updated the location of that particular dollar bill. One example of a bill that traveled widely was one that passed through five states in four years and was last seen in Athens, Greece. The next time you spend some cash and consider where that money might have been, you may want to wash your hands.

Another analysis of paper money, this time in India, discovered that the banknotes harbored pathogenic microbes such as virulent *E. coli*, which causes diarrhea; *Klebsiella*, which can cause mouth, skin, and intestinal diseases; and *Streptococcus*, which can cause strep throat, meningitis, and bacterial pneumonia. Five hundred samples (from five rupee to five hundred rupee denominations) were collected from various sources, such as roadside vendors, butchers, fish mongers, and street sweepers. The authors speculate that so many infectious microbes were found because of the large number of people handling the bills, as well as the damp Indian climate, which could help bacteria survive on such surfaces. "We recommend not shuffling the notes using spit," concluded the authors. "It is also recommended to wash the hands after frequent handling of notes before any hand to mouth operation."[32] This study is similar to that done in Ohio, except that the number of hazardous microbes was higher, perhaps because of the endemic diseases in Indian communities, as well as the practice of shuffling paper currency using spit-moistened fingers.

A Dutch group wanted to determine if the banknote paper that is used to make currency in different countries would vary in its ability to harbor bacteria. Paper money is made of cotton fiber, mixed together in some instances with other fibers, and treated with chemicals such as gelatin to make it more durable. In addition, artificially produced polymers (plastics) are used by some countries to make bills, as they can be designed with special security features that are hard to counterfeit. Romania, Israel, and Malaysia are examples of countries using such bills. Methicillin-resistant *Staphylococcus aureus* (MRSA), Vancomycin-resistant *Enterococci* (VRE), and a multidrug-resistant *E. coli* strain were used in this study to contaminate U.S. dollar bills, Canadian dollar bills, Indian rupees, Moroccan dirhams, Romanian leus, Croatian kunas, and European euros. When the banknotes were tested, both U.S. and Canadian dollars harbored MRSA, the euros harbored *E. coli*, but the Croatian luna remained free of all three strains of bacteria. The Romanian leus, however, harbored and yielded all three pathogens. It is possible, since leus are made of artificial plasticlike material, that they are more hospitable to bacteria. It is important to know what kind of bills bind and harbor more germs and which remain relatively germfree. If it is possible to produce bills that harbor fewer microbes, it may reduce the risk of disease transmission in populations using those currencies.[33] In light of this study, it is a good idea to wash your hands after handling money.

Reservoirs of Pathogens
Rings, Watches, and Stethoscopes

While I have tremendous respect for medical doctors and other medical professionals, it is always productive and beneficial to learn how medical practice can be improved. Previously we discussed a case in which a surgeon's contaminated rings led to wound contaminations and patient infections.[34] A Turkish study confirmed that nurses who wear rings had significantly higher bacterial counts on their hands compared with nurses who did not wear rings. It did not seem to matter whether the rings were plain wedding bands or more elaborate rings set with stones. Even when the nurses cleansed their hands with alcohol-based hand rub, the ring wearers had more bacteria.[35] As a result of these and similar findings, policies have changed in many hospitals, and surgeons are expected to remove all jewelry to reduce the risk of contamination.

The British Department of Health recommended in 2008 that doctors not wear watches, jewelry, or use fake nails, in a "bare below the elbows" dress code, as they can increase the risk of contaminating patients. In India, *Staphylococcus aureus* was found on the hands of 64 percent of healthcare workers who wear watches, compared with 36 percent of those who don't.[36] Some doctors challenged the ban on wristwatches, as they need to use a watch to calculate heart and breathing rates. While it makes sense for surgeons, who make incisions in their patients, to have jewelry-free hands and arms, some argue that other physicians may not need such restrictions, at least with regard to watches.[37]

Just about anything that doctors touch can be a source of germs that can transfer to patients. The badges and lanyards worn by doctors and nurses are hanging off their necks or belts all day and may be picking up microbes from many sources. At Monash Medical Centre in Australia that was indeed shown to be the case, and of the seventy-one healthcare workers who were tested, twenty-seven lanyards and eighteen badges were found to harbor pathogens, including methicillin-resistant *Staphylococcus aureus* (aka MRSA).[38] In particular, dangling equipment is hazardous, as it can swipe across surfaces and pick up germs.

Stethoscopes, which dangle about the neck and are in direct contact with patients, were also found to pick up germs. In one case, the stethoscope picked up MRSA from a patient, after a single medical exam.[39] Doctors' hands as well as their stethoscopes were found to be contaminated, which is not surprising given that physicians typically handle their stethoscopes with their hands and press them up against the patients' chests, backs, or clothing. While stethoscopes are necessary pieces of equipment that doctors typically carry from patient to patient, they should keep them as sanitized as possible. Dr. Dennis Maki of the University of Wisconsin School of Medicine and Public Health goes so far as to recommend using dedicated stethoscopes—that could be well sanitized between patients—for all intensive care unit patients, and perhaps even for all hospitalized patients.[40]

While stethoscopes are essential, stethoscope covers are not. Some medical personnel like to jazz up their stethoscope, since they walk around all day with it draped over the neck. A soft fabric cover was designed to personalize and decorate the stethoscope, and protect the neck of the clinician from rubbing against the stethoscope tube. However, in a Sarasota, Florida, hospital where some clinicians used stethoscope covers, they found pathogenic bacteria such as *Klebsiella* and *E. coli* also decorating the stethoscope covers. In their report, the researchers referred to stethoscope covers as "The Velveteen Rabbit of Health Care," after the popular 1922 children's book by Margery Williams. In *The Velveteen Rabbit*, a rather ordinary stuffed rabbit became the beloved toy of a little boy. When the child developed scarlet fever, the doctor said regarding the stuffed animal, "Why, it's a mass of scarlet fever germs! Burn it at once."[41] (The toy rabbit, who had longed to become a real rabbit, did in the end escape the bonfire and was granted his wish, scampering off into the garden.) While the stethoscope covers are soft and cute, they can be used for years and are rarely, if ever, laundered. Just as in the children's book, it would be good advice to burn them before they spread disease.[42]

Dirty Talking
Cell Phones

Think of the most personal item you own, one that you may touch and hold throughout the day, bringing it wherever you go. You keep it close to your body. It may be the first thing you touch in the morning and the last thing you touch at night. You bring it to meals, into your car, to class or your job, and into the bathroom. If you could, you might shower with it, but that is highly inadvisable. I am talking about your cell phone, of course. A cell phone, almost never out of your reach, is covered with microbes. Think about that the next time you are tempted to borrow someone's phone, or when one is handed to you for you to take a call. It's almost as bad as borrowing someone's toothbrush, which you just wouldn't do. Come to think of it, it might be worse than borrowing a toothbrush, as the toothbrush gets rinsed after each use and has all night to dry out and lose some of those germs.

Mobile communication devices, including cell phones and tablets, are potential reservoirs of infectious agents.[43] That means that they can harbor and transfer germs from one person to another. In a healthcare setting, that could be disastrous and deadly. The number of publications in medical journals regarding cell phones increased exponentially in the first decade of the new millennium. In the 1990s there were only a handful of papers on cellular phones in healthcare settings; there were about 50 published papers in 2002, about 150 in 2004, and almost 350 in 2007, showing how the explosive spread of cell phone use also has increased concern about cell phone contamination. A review article of fifteen studies on contaminated cell phones in healthcare settings revealed that between 9 and 25 percent of the devices are contaminated with pathogenic bacteria. The variation in results reflects the fact that the fifteen studies were conducted using a variety of approaches, in different kinds of healthcare settings, and in a wide range of countries (United States, Canada, United Kingdom, Israel, India, Austria, Turkey, and Barbados). The authors of the review also discuss approaches for reducing risk to patients, by restricting the use of cell phones in healthcare settings (should they be permitted at all in operating rooms, ICUs, or burn units?), enlightening staff about risks, providing hand-hygiene guidelines, and decontaminating the phones.[44]

A more recent study that compared healthcare workers' smart phones and non-smart cell phones reported that about one-fifth of non-smart phones, compared to more than a third of smart phones tested harbored potentially pathogenic bacteria.[45] Smart phones have become integrated into healthcare practice and are used even more than non-smart phones ever were, for communication (e.g., talking and texting) as well as to access data. Smart phones are handled more than non-smart phones, so they could be more of a risk for transmitting germs and, indeed, do appear to collect more dangerous microbes. iPads and other tablets are also more commonly used in clinical settings to manage patient data and could pose risks. In a North Dakota study, twenty hospital iPad screens were tested, and three of them were positive for MRSA. The researchers also showed that iPads can be easily contaminated with MRSA or *C. difficile*, both of which cause nosocomial infections. A moist cloth, alcohol swab, or bleach wipe can cleanse the screen of MRSA; but *C. difficile* is much harder to eradicate, and only bleach works against that pathogen.[46] However, bleach may not be practical, as it may damage sensitive electronic devices.

These devices can carry germs from one person to another, and in a clinical setting this can have very serious implications. In everyday life contaminated devices can also expose us to germs and transmit them from place to place, making us sick. Now that we live in a culture where cell phone use is pervasive, it will be difficult to get people to agree to restrict usage, even though some of these findings indicate that lives may be at stake. So what are we to do with those germ-laden slabs we keep in our pockets, purses, and next to our dinner plates?

First, as we have demonstrated throughout this book, it is a good idea to keep your hands clean and to use proper hand hygiene, in particular after using the bathroom and before eating or touching your mouth, nose, eyes, or other apertures of your body. If you follow this advice, your personal mobile device may not be too contaminated. Nevertheless, it is a good idea to wipe it down on a regular basis with a moist microfiber cloth, like the kind used to clean eyeglasses, as that removes many germs. Some microbes are particularly resilient; *C. difficile*, which are bacteria that form spores, may require bleach, and the influenza virus may require alcohol for removal. But the sensitive nature of our phones and other devices may preclude wiping them off with those strong antimicrobial agents.

Note, however, that there are numerous products that can be purchased to clean these devices. Bausch and Lomb makes Clens, which is dilute (12 percent) isopropyl alcohol, mixed with a common detergent called sodium lauryl sulfate and a small amount of dipropylene glycol methyl ether (or DPM, a solvent used in paints, dyes, inks, brake fluid, and other products). For about twenty dollars, you can buy a kit containing two ounces of the Clens spray cleaner, six premoistened tissues, and a microfiber cleaning cloth. iKlear (also about twenty dollars for a kit) is another product for cleaning electronic devices, which is alcohol-free and has "proprietary ingredients," according to the federal government's requisite material safety data sheet. It is 99.1 percent water, with a small amount of methyl paraben and, presumably, other secret ingredients that do not have to be disclosed because of patent protection. Wireless Wipes, an alcohol-based sanitizer, is another option for cleaning cell phones; the wipes can be purchased for five dollars for a pack of twelve towelettes. It appears that the developer of this product has a unique vision, and probably a sense of humor, as they come in three scents: rosemary peppermint, pomegranate citrus, and green tea cucumber. The company's slogan is "no more dirty talk."

Some tech experts recommend using a homemade concoction of one part 70 percent isopropyl alcohol mixed with one part distilled water to clean cell phones or tablets. Both ingredients are readily available in drugstores and are very cheap.[47] If you go on the Internet, there are lively discussion groups trading advice on how best to keep your electronics shiny and clean. Some recommend dilute soap and water, some say vinegar and water, and some swear by alcohol and water. One recommendation is to use water, alcohol and soft soap, a combination that is similar to the Clens product.

Another way to reduce the bacterial contamination on cell phones is by using ultraviolet (uv) radiation. Ultraviolet radiation penetrates the cell walls of bacteria and disrupts their DNA, killing most living cells. I have never gone so far as to use uv to decontaminate my belongings, but presumably there are people who use the PhoneSoap Charger (about $60), which is a small case designed to fit one smart phone. It has a charging port and uv lightbulbs that irradiate your cell phone to sanitize it. Violife makes uv devices to clean toothbrushes and other items. Some of the Violife devices are in the shape of cute animals, no doubt to encourage children to deposit their toothbrushes in them after use. The Cellblaster is another version ($110), and WOPUTUO makes a $20 uv device that can sanitize cell phones, mp3 players, earbuds, Bluetooth headsets, hearing aids, and any other small objects that fit into the chamber. Come to think of it, in light of all we have discovered about fomites, maybe we should put our finger rings into uv chambers each night.

Food Safety
Food Fomites

Huge books have been written about food safety, and much of that topic is beyond the scope of this book on hand hygiene. But there are relevant issues that we should be aware of regarding the handling of food that may help to keep us healthy.

It is important to keep in mind that most of us do not contract food poisoning most of the time, since we have protective mechanisms built into our bodies. The food we consume is not sterile. Even if we ate right out of the cooking pot, the act of opening the pot lid is enough to introduce microbes into the food. Of course, most microbes are not pathogenic and will not cause disease. But even pathogenic germs do not always cause disease, as the body can resist many types of infection—in part thanks to natural immunity barriers, such as stomach acid that sterilizes food upon contact. In general, in order to make us sick, microbial contamination needs to reach a certain threshold, and food that is well prepared and stored will have a minimal level of contamination.

Food can serve as a fomite—an infected surface, picking up germs from various sources such as contaminated hands, dirty kitchen counters, dishware or utensils, or spores in the air. Raw foods, including fruits and vegetables and uncooked meats, poultry, and eggs, can harbor microbes from the farm, processing facility, or slaughterhouse. That is why it is best practice to wash hands with soap, before food preparation or eating, and again after handling raw meats, poultry, or eggs. Gloves are useful in some circumstances, especially for professional food handling, but they are not essential for day-to-day food preparation in the home as long as you wash your hands properly. If you do use gloves, be sure they are changed on a regular basis, and be cautious that they do not themselves become vectors to transfer germs. For instance, be careful not to touch cooked foods after touching raw meat, poultry, or eggs, and keep raw meat, poultry, or eggs separate from the food you are about to serve.

Since food is not sterile, whatever microbes are found in the food may be able to multiply, given the appropriate conditions. Keeping food refrigerated will inhibit, or slow down, bacterial growth. Keeping food frozen will arrest cell activity, so bacteria will not reproduce. It is important to minimize the amount of time food is kept at room temperature or luke-warm. The longer food sits at a lukewarm temperature, the higher the risk that any contaminating microbes will be able to reproduce, and higher numbers of microbes can overwhelm our body's defenses and make us sick. The key is, unless you are eating it, keep food either very cold (in storage) or very hot (as it is cooked).

Produce can pick up contaminants from the environment. Contaminated water might have been used to irrigate crops or to rinse off the harvested fruits or vegetables. That is how we get outbreaks of *E. coli* that are spread to wherever the produce ends up. It is essential to wash fruits and vegetables very well, as we usually have no idea what corner of the world they came from and how they were handled. Keep in mind that travelers abroad are typically cautioned not to eat fresh fruits and vegetables, as the foreign flora (microbes) can wreak havoc with visitors' digestive tracts (e.g., Montezuma's revenge in Mexico). In one account of traveler's diarrhea in India, *New York Times* correspondent Gardiner Harris admits to eating a just-picked mango in New Delhi, skin and all. If only he had washed the fruit or peeled it, he would have saved himself days of suffering.[48]

Nowadays, foreign fruits and vegetables are in U.S. markets, and we bring them into our kitchens and routinely eat them. It is best practice to wash all the produce you consume. In addition, since factory farming can lead to safety issues with regard to poultry, meat, and eggs, and those foods can be repositories of dangerous microbes,[49] it is wise to keep the raw ingredients separate from other foods, clean any surfaces or utensils used to handle them, and make sure they are thoroughly cooked.

Germs Away from Home
Travel Tips

The discussion on food safety is a good segue to hygiene issues related to travel. After all, as pointed out previously, much of our food comes from other parts of the world or other areas in the United States and has traveled to us over long distances. So we do not need to travel to encounter foreign microbes.

In the United States we pride ourselves on cleanliness, hygiene, and smelling good. The effort to stay clean drives a multibillion-dollar industry, including corporate giants such as Proctor & Gamble, Johnson and John-son, Unilever, and Colgate-Palmolive. However, we all live in a broader in-ternational, global civilization, with people constantly on the move from place to place and country to country carrying germs on and in their bodies and belongings. Germs transported by people in planes, trains, automo-biles, and ships make their way around the world in record time. Although in modern times we have an understanding of germ theory, how microbes are transmitted, and how to reduce the risk of infections, the approaches and attitudes toward hygiene, in particular handwashing throughout the world, vary widely. There are places abroad that share similar values and practices to the United States with regard to hand hygiene. But in some developing countries, frequently because of the lack of basic resources such as adequate drinking and washing water, there are lower standards of hand hygiene and other hygiene practices, which could significantly in-crease the risk of infection, disease, and death.[50] In some regions, however, culture and practice may lead to better hygienic standards. For instance, handshakes are not part of the local culture in Japan, and avoiding hand-shakes likely reduces the risk of infection for natives as well as for travelers.

Since we live in a global society where people travel widely, transport-ing germs along with themselves and their luggage, it is important to be aware of the status of infectious diseases and hygienic behavior around the globe. The 2014 Ebola crisis had Americans on edge, since healthcare workers and others who traveled to Ebola hotspots in Africa were capable of importing that deadly virus across the ocean. Indeed, some people did bring Ebola back to the United States, were deathly ill, and were treated in our American hospitals, and two people died. (Over ten thousand have died so far in Africa.) The Ebola crisis stirred up an American media frenzy of not quite panic, but tremendous concern. This type of international health crisis should raise awareness about healthcare deficiencies in de-veloping countries, and this may affect attitudes about the safety of world travel.

There have been numerous studies on handwashing practices world-wide and their effect on health. One review article collected data from forty-two different studies of handwashing with soap and its effects on the incidence of diarrhea. These studies were conducted by researchers in nineteen different countries. The overall picture is bleak, as the data confirm that most of the world population is far behind in hygiene practices. "From the 42 studies reporting handwashing prevalence we estimate that approximately 19% of the world population washes hands with soap after contact with excreta (i.e., use of a sanitation facility or contact with children's excreta)."[51] That means that worldwide, on average four out of five people fail to wash with soap after contact with human waste. The mean prevalence of handwashing with soap ranged from a low of 5 percent in Tanzania to a high of 72 percent in New Zealand. China had a 13 percent rate, India 15 percent, the United States 49 percent, the Netherlands 50 percent, and the United Kingdom a 52 percent mean prevalence of handwashing with soap. Thus, according to this review article, the practice of handwashing with soap in the United States is roughly equivalent to other developed countries such as the United Kingdom and the Netherlands, but not as impressive as New Zealand. The fact that only half of the U.S. population washes with soap after using the bathroom is not encouraging. Clearly we should do better than that. The countries that ranked significantly lower in handwashing with soap were typically low- and middle-income countries in Africa, the Americas, Southeast Asia, and the Western Pacific region. With regard to planning travel, it may be useful to know how your destination ranks with regard to hygiene, so you can plan and act accordingly in order to stay as healthy as possible.

We demonstrated in chapter 1 that each person has a unique microbiome, each house has its own microbiome, and each subway station has a distinctive microbiome. Naturally, when traveling we encounter different environments with different microbiomes. It is important to protect ourselves when traveling since travelers may be more vulnerable to microbes, particularly if they are novel and are strains of germs not previously encountered. Our immune system develops the ability to protect us from a wide range of microbial challenges. But new germs may escape surveillance and lead to disease.

There are extreme and disturbing examples in history in which explorers and new settlers imported new microbes that transmitted diseases to indigenous populations, thereby decimating them. There is documentation of devastating disease, including smallpox epidemics brought by Europeans, which wiped out vast numbers of Native Americans in North America. The Aborigines in Australia suffered a similar fate when European settlers brought European diseases to that continent. These examples underscore the tremendous impact microbes have had on human history, as well as the importance of our immune system that, by previous exposure, helps us to resist domestic diseases.

When traveling to new areas, it is a good idea to find out if the region has extraordinary risks for particular infectious diseases. In many parts of Africa, South America, and Asia, yellow fever, malaria, hepatitis A, and typhoid present special risks. Travelers can be vaccinated or take medication to dramatically reduce the risk of contracting those diseases. For instance, before a recent trip to South Africa, Zimbabwe, and Botswana, I was vaccinated against hepatitis A and typhoid and took malarone to protect against malaria. The CDC maintains a website that has current information on disease risks for travelers in each country. You simply enter your destination, and it will advise you what vaccines, if any, are needed and how to reduce the risk of contagious diseases while traveling.[52]

Foreign travel, and even domestic travel, can pose challenges in the form of germs encountered in hotels, restaurants, airports, planes, trains, and buses, and public gathering places. Seasoned travelers try to stay in reputable hotels or motels, to minimize the risk of exposure to other people's germs. To improve the chance of clean accommodations, it is advisable to check Internet reviews, as they provide the opportunity to preview facilities and get an idea of the cleanliness and service in hotels and restaurants. Although Internet reviews are not entirely reliable, many travelers will rate their experiences, and this can provide some insight into the quality of a hotel.

Years back, traveling was fraught with hazards, and fleabag hotels really did have fleas, or worse. The Texas bedsheet law of 1907 was one of the first attempts to set standards of cleanliness in hotels. It was approved after a six-foot-eight-inch Texan was frustrated in a hotel where the sheets were too short to cover him from head to toe.[53] The newspaper article reporting this noted, "If there is a bed in a hotel or boarding house in Texas that is equipped with a sheet of shorter length than nine feet the keeper of the hostelry is liable to arrest and heavy fine."[54] The nine-foot sheet law was subsequently passed in Oklahoma in 1908 to combat the spread of tuberculosis.[55] It was designed to ensure that lodgers would have a clean sheet covering the whole bed, so they would not be exposed to germs from previous travelers. A North Dakota law stipulated "that hotels charging fifty cents a night or more shall always change sheets and pillow slips after a guest departs."[56] (For less than fifty cents, lodger beware.)

Travel expert Jill Schensul, who writes for the *Record* of northern New Jersey, has practical tips for travelers to reduce the risk of exposure to germs. She notes that today airplanes have quick turnarounds and are unlikely to have been well cleaned between flights. That means germs from the previous passengers are likely to be left behind, including on the pillows, blankets, tray table, armrests, bathrooms, and so on. Schensul recommends that alcohol-based sanitizer (pack three ounces or less, in order to pass through security) be used to wipe down any surface you will be touching. According to her research, people have been known to actually change their infants' diapers on tray tables. Digest that fact as you are enjoying your airline meal. Schensul also indicates that you should not touch anything in the seatback pocket, as people stash all sorts of disgusting things there (dirty diapers, used vomit bags, to name a few).[57] I would add that some people bring their own pillow and blanket for long flights. That has become more common now that airlines have cut back on amenities of that sort.

With regard to your hotel room, Schensul notes, "You may not have the cleanest house on the planet, but at least you know where the germs come from. You never know who has stayed, slept, bled, partied, spit, barfed and whatevered in your room before you got there."[58] (Her column is probably rated G or PG, so use your imagination for "whatevered.") Staying in a more expensive hotel does not ensure that the room is free of germs. Hotspots that could be most contaminated are those surfaces that are handled or touched most by people, and they could include the bedspread, TV remote, water glasses, doorknobs, faucet handles, and the telephone. Schensul says you should bring antibacterial wipes or spray and wipe down the remote, doorknobs, handles, and phone. Take the bedspread off the bed and put it somewhere out of the way so you do not have to touch it again.[59]

The water glasses that seem clean and shiny can harbor all sorts of surprises. Schensul recommends washing them in hot water for at least two minutes before use, or use disposable cups, if available. Run the shower before you step in, and wear flip-flops to protect feet from shower germs. Do not walk around the hotel room in bare feet. Check the sheets for hairs, bedbugs, or other signs of contamination. Bring and use your own pillow-case. If you are in a place where the water is suspect, drink only bottled water. Brush your teeth and rinse your toothbrush with bottled water; avoid ice cubes and fruits and vegetables washed with water; and keep your mouth closed when showering.[60]

Jill Schensul's rules of traveling sound suspiciously like my father's; perhaps we are related. With regard to restrooms, whether it is a pit in the ground in Thailand or at the Ritz in Paris, Jill applies her "Golden Rule of Filthy Places," namely, "Touch nothing. Everything is suspect." She never flushes a toilet with her naked hand. She tries to never touch banisters. She wipes down surfaces with alcohol-based hand rub, wipes, or spray, similar to what I learned as a child. And she considers these acts "neurotic behaviors that have kept me safe from disease when I travel."[61] She is a germaphobe to be proud of.

I admit that I do not adhere to all of the travel advice offered by Jill Schen-sul, but it is gratifying to discover a like-minded person, a travel authority, who writes from her vast experience. And it is nice to know that there are people out there who are even more vigilant about germs than I am.

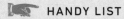 **HANDY LIST**

How to Use Gloves Properly

1 Take a clean pair of gloves for each task.
2 Complete the task.
3 Remove one glove by grabbing the palm and stripping off the glove, taking care to touch only dirty surface to dirty surface.
4 Roll the dirty glove into a ball and hold it in the palm of the other gloved hand.
5 Use the clean hand to pull from under the cuff of the second glove, in the process inverting the glove and turning it inside out. The balled glove should end up inside the second (inverted) glove.
6 Discard the dirty gloves in a step-on garbage receptacle.
7 Wash hands with soap and water. Dry thoroughly.

Source: Health and Safety in the Child Care Setting: Prevention of Infectious Disease: A Curriculum for the Training of Child Care Providers, mod. 1, 2nd ed. (Oakland, CA: California Child Care Health Program, 2001), 37. http://www.ucsfchildcarehealth.org /pdfs/Curricula/idc2book.pdf.

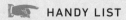

Tips for Staying Healthy When You Travel

1. When flying, wear socks, so if you are required to take off your shoes for airport security, you will not be barefoot.
2. During the security screening, put your cell phone, watch, and other personal items in a Ziploc bag, as they are placed into the same bins as everybody's shoes.
3. When renting a car, wipe down the steering wheel before driving.
4. In airplanes, wipe down or cover surfaces that you will touch with your hands or the back of your head or hair. Bring your own pillow and blanket. Lately I have not had a problem with communal airline blankets, as some airlines seem to have stopped providing them altogether, although some airlines still provide blankets in plastic bags, claiming they are sanitized.
5. In hotel rooms, wipe down the surfaces most likely to be touched by others. Alcoholize the toilet seat, telephone, and remote control, and do not use the end piece of toilet paper that has been artfully folded into a triangle. The person who thoughtfully did that may have just cleaned the toilet and then touched the paper. Throw that end piece away.
6. Many people enjoy traveling because they like the opportunity to experiment with new kinds of exotic foods. I am not one of those people. But if you do this, try to eat those foods in reputable and clean food establishments, and when necessary, stay away from fresh, unpeeled fruits and vegetables, and stick to bottled water.
7. Wash your hands often when traveling, especially after using the bathroom, before eating, and after handling money.
8. If you visit a zoo or other animal facility, wash your hands when you leave and before eating.

Solutions
Protecting Ourselves and Society

In previous chapters I presented many examples of how hand-hygiene practice is terribly important but can be woefully inadequate. Based on this evidence, you may already find yourself being more aware of germs and washing your hands more often and more meticulously. However, as you observe and discuss these issues with others, you will learn that many people still do not appreciate the fact that in order to reduce the risk of infection and disease, hands need to be washed with soap at critical times of the day. About 20 percent of humans worldwide wash their hands with soap after toileting.[1] That leaves 80 percent who do not. The good news is that Americans do much better than the worldwide average, but the bad news is that despite all the hygiene products Americans have available, including pharmacy and supermarket aisles filled with dozens of types of body washes, liquid soaps, and bar soaps of tremendous diversity (e.g., lavender oatmeal soap with goat's milk), only half of Americans wash with soap after going to the bathroom,[2] and only 10 percent of male college students and 7 percent of female college students wash up before eating.[3] These numbers seem rather bleak. How can we improve the hand-hygiene practice of the general public?

More bad news regarding hygiene is that the incidence of hospital-acquired infections attributable to *C. difficile* almost doubled between 2001 and 2008, from 4.5 per thousand adult discharges to 8.6 per thousand. More recent statistics report good news, namely, that the rate of infection declined slightly between 2008 and 2010, dropping to 8.2 per thousand.[4] In recent years, hand hygiene has become an important issue in hospitals, and more resources are being directed toward that issue. Hand hygiene in health care was addressed in chapter 3, and there is good news about formal programs and initiatives that are under study and being developed to improve our attitudes, knowledge, and behaviors with regard to hand hygiene. Additional solutions for healthcare hygiene will be discussed in this chapter.

There are extraordinary challenges in implementing change in hygiene practices, but the good news is that researchers have learned a lot about best practices in hygiene for homes, the community, schools, and medical settings. Most important, evidence-based medicine, which utilizes a scientific approach to solve health-related problems, is making strides in improving hygiene in clinical settings. The scientific approach provides us with the tools to improve healthcare outcomes, and this can lead to rational, evidence-based changes in policy and the practice of medicine. For instance, after many years of surgical scrubbing using traditional protocols, many surgical departments are open to the use of alcohol-based hand-rub protocols, as they have proven to be as effective in disinfecting hands before surgery.[5] This is based on empirical evidence that a double application of alcohol is at least as good in reducing hand contamination as traditional handwashing. In addition, new studies support similar changes in policy for food handlers.[6]

Change in the culture, policy, and practice with regard to hygiene is needed to improve community and personal health, and change is possible through a variety of approaches:

1 *Methods of assessment* help us to measure and record what people are actually doing. Much of this book has addressed the issues of hand hygiene from the perspective of what people are doing, or not doing, about hygiene in clinical settings and in everyday life. We must continue to assess what goes on in hospitals and clinics, classrooms, and the home.

2 *Educational approaches* have been developed to inform people about what works in hand hygiene to improve health outcomes.

3 Behavioral change is difficult, but there are programs that focus on *behavior modification*, as well as appealing to emotions (disgust, embarrassment, shame, pride) to accomplish the goals.

4 Other programs focus on developing *new standard operating procedures* for hand hygiene, to organize and standardize procedures.

5 *Technology* has been developed to monitor and guide behavior.

These five areas are explored in this chapter, and some simple and more complex solutions for improving hand hygiene are offered and encouraged.

The Handshake
Hand-to-Hand Contact

Since changes in hand hygiene are needed, which changes are feasible, and which are unlikely or impractical? One example of a change that could make a difference is banning the handshake in healthcare facilities.[7] Banning handshaking entirely would be extreme, but there is evidence that hand-to-hand contact does, indeed, transfer pathogens. Leila Given, a registered nurse of great vision, was one of the first to discuss the risks posed by handshaking in her 1929 essay, "The Bacterial Significance of the Handshake." In her essay she was clearly distressed by the ignorance or indifference of a woman with a severe head cold, whom she observes sneezing in her hand and then offering the same hand in a handshake.[8] A 1947 medical study dramatically revealed the hazards of handshakes, showing that handshakes can transmit hemolytic streptococci from infected people who had just blown their noses to other individuals.[9]

A more recent study, however, which tested the hands of fourteen school officials who shook 5,209 hands while officiating at a variety of graduation ceremonies in central Maryland, suggested that handshakes actually are not that hazardous. Handshakes do, indeed, transfer microbes, but not all microbes are harmful. On the postgraduation hands, nonpathogenic, harmless bacteria were found in 93 percent of specimens tested, and only two of the samples taken from two of the fourteen school officials had *Staphylococcus aureus*. One sample was found on a right hand and one on a left hand. The researchers suggested that the left-hand contaminant was not picked up from a handshake, since all handshakes were done right-handed; perhaps it was from another surface, such as a contaminated lectern or diploma. Therefore, the presence of only one contaminant of concern on one right hand led the investigators to suggest that the risk of acquiring pathogenic bacteria by handshake at a graduation is one out of 5,209 (or a 0.019 percent probability of acquiring a pathogen per handshake).

That rate of contamination seems surprisingly low, but it is important to consider the parameters of the study, namely, that the people involved in the study were generally healthy. Children and young adults who have serious infectious diseases would not typically attend graduation. In addition, the authors address other limitations of the study. For instance, it is possible that pathogens from earlier handshakes are rubbed off by later handshakes. An even more important limitation is that the study tested only for bacterial pathogens, not viral pathogens, such as the influenza virus and the myriad viruses that can cause the common cold.[10] Many studies show that handwashing reduces the risk of respiratory and other infections, many of which are caused by viruses.[11]

Thus, the graduation study, which only focused on bacterial pathogens, should not reduce the vigilance regarding hand hygiene for anyone who has to shake hands with a lot of people. Remember, it only takes one handshake with one contagious person to expose oneself to disease. Many politicians, members of the clergy, and people in the business world who shake a lot of hands have learned to protect themselves from hand-transmitted germs by using hand sanitizer. School officials also understand that events such as graduations expose them to many hands and germs. In fact, one school official who was asked to participate in the graduation study declined, as his practice during graduation is to discreetly use hand sanitizer every few minutes during the diploma and handshaking ceremony, and he did not want to abandon that practice to participate in the study. It is also important to keep in mind that the graduation scenario is not comparable to a healthcare setting, where there is a much higher risk of contact with infectious diseases and, in particular, drug-resistant microbes.

In another study, researchers compared the transfer of bacteria from one hand to another via three different types of contact greetings: a handshake, a high five and a fist bump. They designed an experiment in which the handshake initiator donned a sterile glove, dipped the glove-covered hand into a liquid culture of nonpathogenic *E. coli* bacteria, and allowed it to dry. A handshake, high-five, or fist bump was completed with a recipient wearing a sterile glove; the recipient's glove was then tested for relative amounts of *E. coli* bacteria. The three types of hand contact were completed by the same pair of subjects five times (using newly prepared gloves each time). Handshaking transferred about twice as many bacteria as a high-five, and about ten times the amount as a fist bump. A prolonged fist bump transferred more bacteria than a brief fist bump. Likewise, a strong handshake transferred about twice as many bacteria as a moderate handshake. The authors note that the handshake has important social and professional value, so it is not likely to be abandoned, but they suggest that the fist bump be adopted as "a simple, free, and more hygienic alternative to the handshake."[12]

During the 2009 H1N1 influenza epidemic, some schools implemented a "no handshaking" policy at graduation. At the University of Michigan, for instance, instead of handshakes they suggested alternative greetings, such as the fist bump, chest bump, and hug. That university has since lifted the ban on handshaking, but they still provide graduates with a choice of greetings. At a recent ceremony, as students lined up to receive their diplomas, many warm hugs, fist bumps, and chest bumps were exchanged.[13] As we have learned, handshakes transfer more germs than fist bumps (although the jury is still out on chest bumps and hugs). Clearly our understanding of hygiene and health has begun to change our culture and behavior, but even small changes in how we interact with each other may lower the risk of spreading infectious disease.

Should handshakes be banned in medical settings? Given that nosocomial infections frequently arise as a result of the transmission of germs from the hands of healthcare workers, and drug-resistant bacteria are a major problem in healthcare settings, changes that might reduce the spread of microbes from person to person in a hospital could save lives. Dr. Mark Sklansky and colleagues at Ronald Reagan UCLA Medical Center in Los Angeles grappled with the question of whether handshaking should be banned from hospitals. They presented the prospect of such a ban as analogous to the ban on smoking in public places. It took decades to convince the public of the health hazards of smoking, to introduce policies to limit smoking in certain venues, and to pass legislation to ensure smoke-free zones. "Removing such a deeply embedded cultural custom from social situations has involved, beyond formal bans/regulations, widespread media and educational efforts, as well as the development and promotion of effective alternatives, such as nicotine gum, in part because of the addictive nature of nicotine."[14] Likewise, handshaking is a "deeply embedded cultural custom" and to remove it from social or professional interactions will require a multipronged approach. To ensure that people understand and adhere to this policy, the authors suggested that signs be posted in appropriate places in hospitals, indicating, "Handshake-free zone: to protect your health and the health of those around you, please refrain from shaking hands while on these premises."[15] They also advised that alternative greetings be devised to replace the handshake. Some examples of contact-free hand gestures suggested by them include the hand wave, the pledge-to-the-flag-style hand over the heart, and the Far Eastern–style bow.[16]

I have noticed that at some formal events (weddings, dinners, and the like), "air kisses" have replaced cheek kisses as a social greeting between women, especially when the greeters do not wish to smudge each other's makeup. Likewise, "air high-fives" or "air fist bumps" could catch on as casual contact-free greetings and provide a way to cordially acknowledge acquaintances, while minimizing the exchange of germs.

Assessment
Measuring Clean Practices

In order to measure behavior and practice, there should be a standardized set of steps in hand-hygiene procedures so that they can be properly monitored. The Centers for Disease Control (CDC) describe the "five simple and effective steps" of handwashing, which they compare to "a do-it-yourself vaccine." The five steps are: "Wet, Lather, Scrub, Rinse, Dry."[17] It would appear that such a simple set of steps is measurable, and that can be useful when assessing hand hygiene in various venues. The World Health Organization (WHO) lists eleven steps of handwashing, as they add specific steps for rubbing and scrubbing hand and finger surfaces with lather. They also direct that the duration of handwashing is at minimum the amount of time it takes to sing the "Happy Birthday" song twice.[18] In addition to the steps directing how hands should be washed, there are lists directing when hands should be washed. The "Five Moments for Hand Hygiene" are listed in the *WHO Guidelines on Hand Hygiene in Healthcare*, defining when and which circumstances in health care demand scrupulous hand hygiene. "Not only does the Five Moments align with the evidence base concerning the spread of HAI [hospital-acquired infections] but it is interwoven with the natural workflow of care and is designed to be easy to learn, logical and applicable in a wide range of settings."[19] The Five Moments are: "(1) Before patient contact. (2) Before an aseptic [sterile] task. (3) After body fluid exposure risk. (4) After patient contact. (5) After contact with patient surroundings."[20] These lists and procedures help to define the task of hand hygiene and permit the behaviors to be monitored and measured.

The World Health Organization's First Global Patient Safety Challenge in 2005 adopted the theme of "Clean Care Is Safer Care." Subsequently in 2009, the campaign "Save Lives: Clean Your Hands" continues their initiative, expanding the WHO's activities and goals. In the current campaign fifty countries are pursuing various projects related to hand hygiene. The list of countries is diverse, with countries from the East and from the West, developed and developing countries, from Bangladesh to Belgium, from Canada to Costa Rica to Croatia, from Ireland to India to Iceland, from Algeria to Vietnam. In the United States a major WHO project with the catchy name of GSI-SC, or "Grime Scene Investigators, South Carolina," has a goal of raising awareness of the importance of clean hands.[21]

Methods for measuring, recording, and analyzing data on hand hygiene are provided in great detail in the more than two-hundred-page monograph prepared by the Joint Commission on "Measuring Hand Hygiene Adherence: Overcoming the Challenges."[22] The Joint Commission is a consortium of the world's leading health organizations, among them the CDC, the WHO, and the National Foundation for Infectious Diseases, who prepared this cleanliness "bible" — a monograph of hand-hygiene assessment. The monograph specifies strategies for measuring hand hygiene, observing the adherence to practices and deciding whom to observe, how to measure compliance, how to conduct surveys, how to evaluate thoroughness of hand cleansing, and how to interpret data. The document opens by raising awareness of the common misconceptions concerning hand hygiene. For instance, they ask whether the following statements are true or false: (1) *"Everybody knows when to clean their hands.* False." They expand on that statement by explaining that most people can carry out personal hand hygiene properly, but hand hygiene related to patient care is much more complicated since, for instance, sometimes one encounter with a patient may require several instances of hand cleansing. (2) *"It is easy to determine whether a person has cleaned his or her hands.* False." Even if someone has washed their hands, it may or may not have been done adequately, and it might have been at the wrong time relative to the risk of contamination. (3) *"People who don't perform hand hygiene when they should are careless or lazy or both.* Usually false." Most health-care personnel care deeply about their patients and want to care for them appropriately. But perfect compliance is unrealistic, as human behavior is inevitably flawed. If the institution is supportive and provides educa-tion, training, and reminders about hand hygiene, as well as the hygiene facilities and materials that are needed, this will improve the outcome. It takes a lot of resources to monitor adherence, and it is expensive in terms of personnel and time. But it is worth it since it reduces the incidence of hospital-acquired infections and improves patient outcomes.[23]

The monograph goes on to explain that major approaches to measur-ing hand-hygiene compliance are by direct observations, by measuring the use of materials (soaps, alcohol-based hand rubs, etc.), and by conducting surveys. It is more reliable to use multiple methods to assess hand hygiene in the institution. The goal is improvement in the performance of person-nel in carrying out hand-hygiene protocols, in order to protect themselves and the patients.[24]

Along with WHO programs and CDC recommendations, the mono-graph has spurred many healthcare centers worldwide to train and moni-tor hand hygiene. Using these types of approaches, the National University Hospital in Singapore instituted a training program, and then evaluated hand-hygiene compliance of 5200 clinical staff. The intervention raised awareness, but the outcome was less than perfect. Despite the fact that the assessment immediately followed training, only 72 percent of staff per-formed at acceptable levels. When handwashing techniques were checked using UV light tests that reveal dirty spots on the hands, there were numer-ous instances where parts of the hands and fingers were not adequately washed. "Nurses performed best (77 percent pass) and women performed better than men (75 percent vs. 62 percent)," reported the authors.[25]

Education

Who should be educated about hand hygiene? In order to reduce the risk of infectious diseases, everyone needs the information, skills, and moti-vation to achieve the appropriate hand-hygiene goals. Education should start in families and schools, with initiatives aimed at children. There are many fine children's books that address the issues of handwashing and health. Unfortunately, those lessons may not be retained through adolescence and adulthood, and inadequate hand hygiene may be the norm for many people.

Healthcare workers, child-care workers, and food handlers require the knowledge, skills, and attitudes regarding hand sanitation to keep patients, children, and patrons safe. There have been many educational and training initiatives, which have some level of success in improving compliance and healthcare outcomes. The diverse approaches used to teach about hand hygiene reflect different philosophies regarding learning. For instance, there are DVDs that provide information on the benefits of hand hygiene and show the methodology. One such video instructs patients on how they can reduce the risk of infections in healthcare facilities. It raises awareness and gives instructions on technique.[26]

A review of forty-five studies on hand hygiene demonstrates the effectiveness of "bundled approaches" to hand hygiene, in other words, using combinations of methods to raise awareness of hand hygiene. The approaches include education, reminders, feedback, administrative support, and access to alcohol-based hand rub.[27] To change ingrained and lifelong behaviors it is likely that many tactics will be necessary.

One web-based program combined a "fully automated intervention" with motivational messages and information on hand hygiene. This intervention used technology to reach, teach, and motivate people to change their behavior. A study on the effectiveness of this intervention was carried out in Southern England in 2010, shortly after the onset of the H1N1 influenza pandemic. It was designed to encourage handwashing as an effective approach in reducing risk of infectious disease, as a socially desirable act, and as something that is easy to do. Subjects participated in four weekly Internet-based sessions. The first session introduced the participants to the medical team, provided information about handwashing and virus transmission, and instructed how and when to wash hands. Subjects were asked to complete a "hand-washing plan," which they were supposed to print out, sign, and post at home for other family members to see and join in. Three additional sessions continued to encourage positive attitudes and the notion that handwashing is a societal norm, and that the act of handwashing is not difficult. The subjects who participated in the Internet intervention demonstrated significantly higher rates of handwashing compared to the control group immediately after the four sessions and even two months later.[28] This program is valuable because once the web-based materials are set up, the intervention is not costly to run and is generally accessible to anyone with Internet access. It is theoretically available to people of different ages and socioeconomic groups. In practice, however, the web-based nature of the intervention may be an obstacle to those who do not have ready access to the Internet, such as people in lower socioeconomic groups or less technology-oriented older adults. Given that we are in a highly web-connected society, it would make sense to continue to develop online programs that provide interventions for hand hygiene.

For smart phone and tablet users, there are hand-hygiene applications ("apps") that provide training on how to wash hands. Bio-RiteAR is a free app that shows the optimal duration of each part of the handwashing process. It also provides knowledge-based statements, such as "Did you know? Bacteria hide under watches and bracelets (there could be as many germs under your ring as there are people in Europe)." The WHO "Five Moments for Hand Hygiene" also are presented in the app.[29]

Another app called HandyMD is a game in which the player takes the role of Dr. Handrew, a character who must wash hands before treating the patient. In the true spirit of video games, as you progress through the levels it becomes more challenging to keep your hands clean. The ubiquitous sink must be visited again and again before treating the patient. When closing the app, the prompt reads: "So, you want to quit. Make sure you clean your hands after playing this game."[30] This may be a good way to reach younger people, who tend to enjoy video games and apps.

An inexpensive approach that can be used in schools teaches children about hand hygiene the old-fashioned way, with "verbal cues" from their actual teacher. In other words, the teacher instructs them to "wash your hands then line up for lunch," followed by the teacher modeling the behavior. A program that used this approach also included an educational session with a guest educator who gave a thirty-minute lesson on germs and sickness, when and how to wash hands, and when to use hand sanitizers. The lesson was followed by the children using a simulated germ solution that allowed them to see how well they did in washing. This can inspire pride in their accomplishment. First graders improved so much that they went from 63 percent to 100 percent compliance by the end of the training. Second graders went up to 94 percent, fifth graders rose from 12 percent to 52 percent, and sixth graders, who did not finish all phases of the program, showed a decrease in compliance from 38 percent to 33 percent.[31] Clearly small children are more malleable and willing to take directions compared to middle-school children, who are typically more challenging to reach and less cooperative. From this data, and from what every parent knows about the middle school and teenage years, in the words of Rogers and Hammerstein, "You've got to be taught before it's too late; before you are six or seven or eight."[32]

Further on the topic of educating children, Dr. Will Sawyer, a self-proclaimed infection-prevention specialist, developed a comic character, Henry the Hand, to teach parents and children about hand hygiene. The website www.HenrytheHand.com features banners proclaiming: "Protect your baby—ask everyone to wash their hands upon entering your home" and "Hand awareness—spread the word, not the germs." Dr. Sawyer's four principles of hand awareness are: "(1) Wash your hands when they are dirty and BEFORE eating. (2) DO NOT cough into your hands. (3) DO NOT sneeze into your hands. (4) Above all, DO NOT put your fingers into your eyes, nose or mouth."[33] The website also offers hand hygiene–related merchandise for sale, such as a Henry the Hand bow tie ($45), a portable sink ($1,200), a training DVD ($100), and the ability to rent a Henry the Hand costume for your class or other group for $240 for two days. The costume is seven feet tall when inflated and comes with a "skit" that can be presented to children's groups. Of course, you need to provide your own actor to wear the costume and play the part.[34] I wonder if anyone has thought of renting it for their child's birthday party. It surely would be the only seven-foot-tall walking and talking hand on the block.

The Yuck Factor: Using Disgust to Save Lives

In my many years of studying and teaching bioethics, I have come to appreciate some of the human motivations that determine what is and is not appropriate behavior. Humans all over the world have different views on some issues related to the human condition. For instance, there are varied norms with regard to the role and status of women in society, and there are different approaches to child rearing. But there are also principles that are fairly universal, for example, the bond between mother and baby, and the taboo against incest with close family members (siblings, parents, children).

One universal human emotion, disgust, helps us to stay healthy by avoiding germ-laden bodily wastes, spoiled food, and other health hazards. In bioethics we refer to the human impulse to reject that which is disgusting or abhorrent as the "yuck factor." Humans and other animals have a strong yuck factor with regard to feces, urine, or contaminated food. For many people, gory and bloody scenes are disgusting. Bodily waste and bloody gore look and smell bad to us and we avoid them. Experts in the field believe that there is a biological basis to these emotions and that disgust is "an adaptation to avoid disease-causing microbes and parasites."[35] It may be biologically determined, although some conditioning is likely to be involved, as babies do not appear to be disgusted by the sight or smell of human waste.

There is compelling evidence that disgust can be used to influence behavior and encourage more healthful choices. In October 2012 pictorial health warning labels began to appear on cigarette packs sold in the United States. The objective was to graphically portray the health risks of smoking with explicit pictures, in order to discourage cigarette smoking. Some of the images used are disgusting pictures of disfiguring disease, such as mouth cancer and lung cancer. Cigarette packs that show "gruesome, diseased organs or human suffering due to smoking" have a greater impact on smokers than text warnings alone, and demand was lower for packs with graphic depictions of disease and human suffering compared with text-only warnings.[36]

Dr. Valerie Curtis, of the London School of Hygiene and Tropical Medicine, has been studying disgust for most of her career and has proposed harnessing disgust to change hand-hygiene behavior. "I suggest that hygiene has biological origins as the set of behaviours that serves to avoid infection, and that it is exhibited by most animals," writes Curtis. "I show that hygiene remains partly instinctive in humans, driven by an innate sense of the need to avoid that which disgusts." She cites observations of behaviors from the lowliest worms up to mammals like us, demonstrating that there is an aversion to diseased animals and germ-laden food. "Does the insight that hygiene behavior is driven not by rationality, but by deep and ancient urges within us, which are not entirely under our conscious control, have any implications for hygiene today?" asks Curtis. While education and appealing to the rational side of the brain may help to convince people to practice good hygiene, she suggests using disgust to improve hygienic practices. In Ghana she helped to develop a campaign encouraging handwashing by "[making] people feel that not washing hands with soap was disgusting." The campaign resulted in a 41 percent increase in Ghanians washing hands with soap.[37]

In "Why Disgust Matters" Valerie Curtis lists twenty-four infectious diseases and their "disgust elicitors" that keep us away from victims and their germs. Diarrheal diseases, caused by bacterial and viral pathogens, are associated with spoiled food and contaminated water, as well as feces. People suffering from measles, plague, and leprosy have disgusting skin lesions and sores that repel others. Individuals with respiratory infections of all sorts exude nasal mucous and may be coughing and sneezing, which would tend to keep others away. "A better understanding of disgust," reasons Curtis, "offers practical lessons that can enhance human flourishing."[38]

Many parents appear to be adept at modeling disgust and teaching young children to avoid disgusting things. They transmit the disgust response to small children on many occasions, such as during diaper changes, toilet training, or during the process of wiping excreta off the wall and carpets after a toddler has divested herself of a dirty diaper. Small children appear oblivious to disgusting sights and smells until they reach the age of two or three. "Facial expression may provide one model for entraining disgust," reported Megan Oaten and coauthors in a study of parents and children. In addition to facial expressions, there are other signals used to communicate disgust such as verbal expressions (words such as "ick," "yuck," and "phew") and gestures of avoidance (looking away, walking away, or covering the offending object). Oaten's group showed that when confronted with something disgusting, parents who instructed their small children to wash their hands also gave more cues related to disgust to the children. "Evidence for parent-child transmission was observed, with parents of younger children in the presence of a disgust elicitor emoting more disgust to their offspring and these children showing the greatest behavioral avoidance of the potential contaminants."[39] The strong emotion of disgust leads to the desire to remove, avoid, or cleanse it away.

If parental disgust works on two-year-olds, maybe the feeling of disgust can be used to change the behavior of adults with regard to germ-laden hands. One group wanted to determine if different messages posted in washrooms would influence handwashing behaviors. The sixteen different messages, flashed on electronic signs in British highway service station restrooms, had a variety of ways to convey a hand-hygiene message. Some were designed to be informative ("Water doesn't kill germs, soap does," or "Washing hands with soap avoids 47% of disease"), or evocative of disgust ("Don't take the loo with you—wash with soap" and "Soap it off or eat it later"). The researchers electronically monitored nearly two hundred thousand restroom uses, concluding that "unobtrusive observation of behavior in a natural setting" can give insight into the best ways to change hand-hygiene behavior. Even though unobtrusive observation of people in bathrooms sounds a bit sketchy, there were some interesting outcomes. Compared to a blank sign, the posting of any message related to hygiene correlated with increased handwashing (although most were not statistically significant increases), with one exception: "Soap adds a fresh touch" was associated with a (not significant) decrease in handwashing in women. Note that women and men reacted differently in a number of instances to the messages, and "Soap adds a fresh touch" correlated with increased handwashing in men (and that increase was statistically significant). The authors observed that knowledge-based posting was most effective for women ("Water doesn't kill germs, soap does), while for men, disgust-based posting ("Don't take the loo with you—wash with soap") had a significant effect. The conclusion? "The gender differences we found suggest that public health interventions should target men and women differently."[40]

Perhaps eliciting feelings of disgust increases handwashing more in children and men than in women because women, who generally handle many disgusting tasks at home, already have a higher baseline and feeling of disgust regarding germ-laden hands. That may be why, in this study, the "disgusting" messages did not significantly increase handwashing for women.

Can we harness the power of other emotions to improve hand hygiene? An Ottawa Hospital Research Institute program sought to apply behavioral theories to improve hand hygiene. The authors lamented that with all of the publications and initiatives on hand hygiene, as well as public health guidelines and policies, many studies show that healthcare workers' compliance still languishes at less than 50 percent, with physicians scoring even lower. Ottawa Hospital implemented a hygiene program that successfully increased physician hand-hygiene compliance from a paltry 14–17 percent (2004–2006) to 65–69 percent in 2011. "In spite of this increase," they noted, "physician compliance continues to lag behind that of most other occupational groups and is below the corporate goal of 80 percent."[41] They wanted to find out what factors were keeping staff from even better performance.

The authors discuss barriers to hand-hygiene compliance and speculate on how to improve the outcomes. Physicians' excuses for not cleansing hands that were discussed in this article included a "high workload or feeling too rushed" and environmental issues such as the lack of soap, broken dispensers, and the lack of paper towels. Additional barriers proposed to explain lower compliance of physicians include that doctors perceive their compliance to be higher than it actually is, the tendency of practitioners to develop "a more cavalier attitude toward infection control as clinical experience increases," that role models for hand hygiene are lacking, and that the "hospital or unit culture vis-à-vis patient safety is inadequate." There is no easy answer to these issues, but based on these problems, the team proposed a study protocol to be carried out in their hospital.[42]

The study conducted by the Ottawa team utilized interviews to collect qualitative data from doctors. Based on in-depth interviews with forty-two "key informants" (randomly selected physicians from subgroups of staff physicians and residents), the participants' answers were categorized into fifty-three "specific beliefs" related to hand hygiene. Many of these beliefs reveal flaws in the medical system. For instance, the beliefs ranged from "I am aware of evidence linking hand hygiene to healthcare-associated infections" (64 percent of respondents) to "I am not aware of evidence linking hand hygiene to healthcare-associated infections" (21 percent). Thirty-six percent of respondents did not think they had training in hand-hygiene practice. Nineteen percent indicated that hand hygiene is difficult to practice. Fourteen percent were not confident that they follow hand-hygiene guidelines, and 33 percent indicated that in an emergency situation they are "less likely to practice hand hygiene." Forty-eight percent revealed that when they are busy they are "less likely to comply with hand hygiene guidelines." Thirty-eight percent agreed that "hand hygiene should be performed by all healthcare professionals." Twenty-six percent thought that "physician hand hygiene compliance is suboptimal." Twenty-nine percent believed they had never been asked by a patient if they had washed their hands.[43]

Granted, these are qualitative data derived from interviews, but after analysis of the fifty-three categories of beliefs, themes and patterns emerge. The authors of the study proposed future interventions that will address deficits in knowledge, provide better training of hygiene skills, remedy the environmental deficits, as well as deal with social and professional issues relevant to healthcare workers.[44] The physicians who were interviewed are on the front lines of medical practice in the hospital, and they articulated much of what was suspected with regard to handwashing by physicians. There are many aspects of healthcare worker hand hygiene in need of attention, and the challenge will be to address issues that encompass all of them.

One thing that concerns me about the Ottawa hospital initiative is that the "corporate goal of 80 percent" still falls far short of universal hand hygiene. Perhaps they were trying to be realistic and to set what they projected to be attainable goals. However, in a more idealistic world, we should strive for the best record possible, and 80 percent is a low B grade in school. We need to set a high bar for hospital hygiene—we should take strides to reach that A.

Simple Solutions

The principle of Occam's razor[45] states that in approaching a problem for which there can be simple, straightforward explanations, or alternatively, more convoluted multidimensional ones, simplest is best. In empirical research it is a good idea to investigate simple solutions even if the problem appears complex. In that spirit, we will consider some simple solutions to the problem of inadequate hand hygiene.

One simple method to increase compliance in healthcare units, institutions, and even private venues is to find the best location for alcohol-based hand-rub stations. And the best way to decide where to place them is to find out where people need the devices. In many stores, hand-rub stations are found near exits. In the zoo, hand-rub stations are placed just outside the children's animal petting area. In hospitals and clinics, one should ask the nurses and doctors where hand-rub stations are needed most and what location makes the most sense. In a study in Rotterdam, the Netherlands, researchers interviewed medical staff members and observed the workflow to determine frequency of use of hand sanitizer stations in different locations; and based on that data, the stations were relocated accordingly. Hand hygiene near the entrance to the room was the top priority; hand-rub dispensers near the computer in the back of the room were less important.[46] This simple, logical, and inexpensive approach can potentially raise compliance, as medical personnel who are rushing will be more likely to sanitize hands if the stations are at their fingertips (no pun intended).

Another simple solution involves focusing more attention on the hand hygiene of patients; this is an area that is often ignored, but which should be a priority. The patients' own hands can be contaminated and can then transfer microbes to and from visitors, healthcare workers, their own skin, wounds or waste products, to other parts of their body. Patients who are bedridden cannot readily wash their own hands because they cannot get to a sink or hand-rub station. One study demonstrated that attention to patient hand hygiene can reduce the incidence of *Clostridium difficile* infections in hospitalized patients.[47] Thus, with a minimal investment, the cleansing of patients' hands, while a simple step, could improve healthcare outcomes.

In fact, as a matter of routine, anyone who is disabled or incapacitated may need assistance with basic hand hygiene, whether or not they are in a hospital. Clearly very young children need assistance with hand hygiene, but elderly people also may need and appreciate help with this task. Failing eyesight may make it difficult for elderly people to see that their hands are soiled, unsteady hands make it hard to wash properly, and difficulty walking can add to the challenge of getting to a sink when needed.

Better Hygiene through Humiliation, Shame, and Technology

Perhaps we could just embarrass people into washing their hands. "Better hygiene through humiliation" describes electronic devices that signal when a healthcare professional has failed to wash hands before approaching a patient. Biovigil is one such system that includes electronic badges, patient room sensors, and a central base station. The approach to improving hand hygiene "aims to exploit a very powerful emotion: shame."[48]

A video describing the Biovigil system reports that "HAIs, or healthcare associated infections, are now the fourth leading cause of death in America and cost the U.S. healthcare system between 30 and 40 billion dollars each year. . . . Two million patients acquire an infection in U.S. hospitals every year and nearly 100,000 people die from them." It goes on to explain, "We know the HAI problem is closely related to hand hygiene, however dozens of studies indicate that hand hygiene compliance is only achieved approximately 50 percent of the time."[49]

The Biovigil motto is, "Hand hygiene monitoring as simple as a traffic light."[50] Each healthcare worker wears a badge that is registered to that worker. The system detects when a healthcare worker enters or leaves a patient's room, hence it is designed to measure compliance with moment 1 and moment 4 of the WHO "My 5 Moments for Hand Hygiene," namely, "before touching a patient" and "after touching a patient." Upon entering a patient's room, the badge chirps and flashes yellow to remind the healthcare worker to sanitize hands. If he or she does not comply, the badge flashes red and emits a warning sound. When hands are sanitized, the sensors in the badge detect alcohol on the user's hands, and the badge turns green. The company explains that the monitoring involves four steps: remind, record, reassure, and report. The device reminds the healthcare worker to sanitize hands; the system records whether or not hands were sanitized; the green light on the badge reassures the patient that the healthcare worker has clean hands; and the data that is collected on each and every worker is reported to the centralized system for analysis. This automated system removes the burden from the patient with regard to asking the doctor or nurse to cleanse hands. Patients in the hospital are typically too sick to notice, or too timid to insist, that their caretakers cleanse hands. The description of the Biovigil system stresses that they are giving patients a sense of safety, and they provide data showing hand-washing compliance results of over 95 percent.[51]

MedSense is another electronic monitoring system designed to measure compliance with moment 1 and moment 4 of the WHO "My 5 Moments for Hand Hygiene." The badges in this system sense proximity to patient beds and to sensors in the soap and alcohol dispensers. A Hong Kong–based study monitored compliance using the electronic system compared with monitoring by an infection-control nurse. During the time that an actual person was watching, compliance was 2.8 times higher than when the electronic devices alone were measuring compliance. This is a classic example of the Hawthorne effect, whereby people perform better as a result of knowing that someone is watching them. A study of industrial productivity done from 1924 to 1932 at the Hawthorne Works, a Western Electric factory near Chicago, revealed that being part of a research study where one is observed could lead to a temporary increase in productivity.[52] During three months of evaluation of seventeen nurses, three physiotherapists, and a healthcare assistant, for almost 14,000 hand-hygiene opportunities, the overall compliance was 35.1 percent. When the infection-control nurse was watching, compliance was 88.9 percent as measured by the electronic system and 95.6 percent as measured by the observer. (The difference between the two measurements may be because of what is registered as a handwashing opportunity by the device versus by the human observer.) When only the electronic devices were used and no one was watching, and nurses shared badges making it impossible to determine individual scores, compliance was measured at 23.7 percent. When no one was watching, but they used individually assigned badges, compliance rose to 34–36 percent.[53] In this case the Hawthorne effect appears to work better when a flesh-and-blood person is observing rather than an electronic device. The authors cite other reports of electronic monitoring showing a wide range of outcomes, as some programs claim to see dramatic increases in compliance with electronic systems, and some show little improvement. They conclude that "further investigation has to be performed to understand if a sustained improvement in hand hygiene practice can be achieved by the use of electronic monitoring systems."[54]

A British study reviewed the effectiveness of nineteen different technologies, including those that used infrared badges, alcohol-detecting badges, radio frequency badges, smart video systems, monitoring based on staff use of water taps, staff use of hand-rub or soap dispensers, thermal sensors, and other designs. The researchers wanted to determine if the technologies are "fit for purpose" (FFP); in other words, are they measuring what needs to be measured vis-à-vis hand hygiene? If we expect hand hygiene to work, healthcare workers have to comply with all of the "WHO 5 Moments for Hand Hygiene," that is, to summarize: (1) Before touching a patient, (2) before any clean/aseptic procedure, (3) after body fluid exposure risk, (4) after touching a patient, and (5) after touching patient surroundings. Their conclusion is that none of the technologies are fit for purpose. They are designed to, at best, evaluate numbers 1 and 2, whether hands have been sanitized before and after patient contact, and for some technologies, after leaving patient surroundings. As for WHO number 2, whether hand hygiene was done before attempting any clean/aseptic procedure, the authors quipped that in order to do this they would need "mind-reading technologies." They noted that "currently such behavior-predicting technologies do not exist, and may never be a feasible option for the clinical environment" and concluded that even if such capabilities were possible, "The question of whether healthcare professionals would engage with 'mind-reading' technologies is doubtful, considering existing hesitancy towards current hand hygiene technologies." Thus, although technologies have the potential to improve the hygiene in hospitals, considering the inability to measure all of the WHO moments for hand hygiene, the authors do not judge the technologies as fully fit for purpose.[55] If the purpose is to ensure that healthcare workers predictably and consistently practice hand hygiene when it is clinically necessary, technology does not fulfill the need. It is way too easy to skip a hand-hygiene moment when it is most needed, that is, right before an aseptic (germfree) procedure, such as changing a catheter or aspirating a ventilator tube.

A simple way to monitor staff compliance, and possibly encourage better hand hygiene, is by measuring the use of hand-hygiene product, either hand soap or alcohol-based hand sanitizer. That approach does not give information on individual use or hygiene practices, but individual members of the team may raise the frequency of hand sanitizing if they know that product usage is being monitored (another example of the Hawthorne effect). It also does not reveal when the hands were sanitized, only whether staff is using more of the cleansing product. One study found that when staff members were aware that hand hygiene was being monitored by the weighing of soap dispenser bags, handwashing rates increased dramatically (up to 400 percent higher).[56] This is an example of using group accountability to encourage handwashing.

Another simple solution is to engage in the ultimate in shame and humiliation by the use of video monitors, which can serve as a Big Brother type of observer. Use of video is a controversial approach and may be, as the title of one article addressing it states, "A step too far."[57] It may, however, be just what the doctor (and nurses) ordered. A most extreme example of this kind of intervention would be the posting of videos on a public website such as YouTube, no doubt an act that would provoke an outcry with regard to privacy issues, and possibly lawsuits.

Standard Operating Procedures

Improvement of hand-hygiene compliance could be accomplished by developing standard operating procedures (SOPs) that better organize the process of patient care. By careful planning, that is, by having all equipment and supplies handy and by preplanning procedures down to the smallest steps, it is possible to reduce the number of hand-hygiene events needed. For instance, if all the materials for a dressing change of a healing incision are conveniently organized, it will reduce the possibility that hands are contaminated between the hand sanitation event and completing the task. Operating rooms are organized in this manner, so that once the staff is scrubbed and gowned, all necessary supplies and equipment are on hand and can be accessed without compromising sterility. With thought and planning, other medical procedures can be executed with equal care.

In the emergency department in a hospital located in Aachen, Germany, SOPs were developed with the goal of improving hand hygiene and healthcare outcome. Flowcharts that were developed for handling intravenous equipment, wound dressing, and the like were prepared and provided on cards for personnel to have handy. Protocols were designed to optimize and standardize invasive procedures, including hand-hygiene moments.

In 378 patient cases, hand-hygiene compliance increased from 21 to 45 percent; and because of better organization and planning, the number of hand rubs necessary for each procedure dropped almost 50 percent. Improving the workflow practices led to more efficient completion of tasks, a reduction in avoidable hand rubs, and a reduction in the number of glove changes needed. "The standardization of workflow may be an appropriate way to improve the overall quality of HH [hand hygiene] and thus increase patient safety." An important outcome was that hand-hygiene compliance improved significantly without increasing the burden of time-intensive tasks for the already overworked staff.[58]

Legislation and Regulation

The United States has a history of legislation that is designed to protect the public, the consumer, children, patients, and communities. While there are federal guidelines on hand-hygiene issues from the Centers for Disease Control[59] that provide advice and models for action, more formal federal codes establish hygiene standards for food establishments as well as nursing homes. It would not be possible to cover all aspects of regulation and legislation relating to hygiene in this book. However, it is worthwhile to comment on the role of codes, regulations, and legislation, as they have made a tremendous impact on the health of individuals and communities.

From the 1907 Texas bedsheet law, in which state legislation first addressed hotel hygiene,[60] to today, federal and local authorities have worked to protect the public from the risks of infectious diseases. An example of an area in which strict legislation has improved healthcare outcomes is in nursing home care. The Federal Nursing Home Reform Act[61] was enacted by Congress in 1987, in response to exposés of inadequacies, malpractice, and mistreatment of nursing home residents. Nursing homes that receive federal Medicare and Medicaid funds are required to comply with certain rules that relate to the residents' physical, mental, and psychosocial well-being. For instance, the facilities are required to have sufficient nursing staff. They are to ensure that residents do not develop bedsores. If they do have pressure sores, the staff are to treat them to prevent infection and to promote healing. There are many other facets to this legislation, and these laws protect many elders and improve their quality of life.

With regard to hygiene, and in particular hand hygiene, food code legislation provides a good example of how the government can protect the public. The Federal Food Code appeared in its first form in 1934, as the Restaurant Sanitation Regulations. Later versions included regulations on "Eating and Drinking Establishments" (1935), food vendors (1957), and retail food stores (1982). The current Food Code first appeared in 1993 and has been revised every few years. The 2013 version is the eighth edition, and it is 768 pages long. It was developed to be "a model for safeguarding public health and ensuring food is unadulterated and honestly presented when offered to the consumer."[62] The development of the most recent edition involved collaboration with the U.S. Department of Agriculture's Food Safety and Inspection Service and the Centers for Disease Control and Prevention of the U.S. Department of Health and Human Services. The intention of this code is to provide a uniform approach to food safety that can be reflected in local statutes, codes, and ordinances. Some of the major goals of this code are to reduce the risk of food-borne illnesses, to provide standards for inspections of food providers, and to establish uniform standards for food safety.[63]

Those sections that relate most to hand hygiene are "Employee Health" and "Personal Cleanliness." The Food Code stipulates that food establishments must follow certain regulations to be granted a permit to operate. Food workers are obligated to disclose when they have infectious diseases or skin conditions, and the permit holder is required to report when food workers have infectious diseases that can potentially be transmitted through food. The code lists a number of symptoms to be further investigated: vomiting, diarrhea, jaundice, sore throat with fever, boils, and infected wounds or lesions on the hands or wrists that cannot be adequately covered and isolated. In addition, if a worker is diagnosed with an illness such as norovirus, *Shigella*, *Salmonella typhi*, or Hepatitis A, or if the worker has a history of exposure to one of those diseases, it must be reported. In the event of infection, under certain conditions, the "person in charge shall exclude or restrict a food employee from a food establishment."[64]

Handwashing is addressed in the Food Code, specifying that "Food employees shall clean their hands and exposed portions of their arms, including surrogate prosthetic devices for hands or arms for at least 20 seconds," using the CDC's five-step procedure. A disposable paper towel should be used to turn off the faucet and open the restroom door to avoid recontamination of washed hands. Hands must be washed immediately before touching food, and after touching any other parts of the skin, after using the bathroom, touching animals, coughing, sneezing, blowing one's nose, eating, drinking, using tobacco, touching raw food, and before putting on protective gloves for food handling. Hand antiseptics that are designated by the FDA as GRAS (generally recognized as safe) may be used if hands are not soiled. Fingernails must be kept trimmed and filed smooth, and no nail polish or artificial nails are permitted unless gloves will be worn. "Except for a plain ring such as a wedding band, while preparing food, food employees may not wear jewelry including [jewelry with] medical information on their arms and hands."[65]

The Federal Food Code was developed to act as a guideline for local codes and laws. One of the most extensive local codes, the New York City Health Code, covers more than sixty areas of concern, including laboratories, drinking water, food and drugs, mobile food vending, animals, tanning facilities, and deaths and disposal of human remains. In the section on "Reportable Diseases and Conditions," there are almost one hundred examples, such as anthrax, cholera, specific strains of *E. coli*, hepatitis, measles, polio, MRSA, typhoid fever, and tuberculosis. The New York City Health Code addresses child day-care regulations, including toileting, handwashing, and diaper changing. The food preparation section of the code is very similar to the Federal Food Code, including the "duty to exclude," which bans employees who are disease carriers from handling food. The "Barber Shop" section requires handwashing with soap and water "before attending a patron and immediately after using the toilet." That section of the code bans the use of a "powder puff, sponge or neck duster" (remember those?) on haircut clients, and any implement used on a patron must be "clean and sanitary."[66]

These codes and laws are effective in keeping us safe in many respects, but they are far from perfect and many hazards still exist. For one thing, verifying compliance with the code can be challenging and takes government personnel and inspectors; the system is inadequate to monitor all facilities. Second, many areas do not fall under the purview of government regulation, and with no oversight, the public may be exposed to unknown hazards. An example of this is the antibacterial chemical triclosan, which has been on the market in many products for years, even though it never received the designation of GRAS (generally recognized as safe), the FDA's seal of approval.

Another example of hygiene-related hazards that have slipped through the cracks of regulation are reusable medical devices. In October 2014, forty-eight-year-old Antonia Torres Cerda died from complications after medical treatment involving a duodenoscope (a type of endoscope used to peer into the small intestine), which was contaminated with deadly bacteria. Six other patients at Ronald Reagan UCLA Medical Center in Los Angeles contracted CRE, a drug-resistant form of Enterobacteriaceae, from the same FDA-approved type of duodenoscope. In March 2015, it was disclosed that four patients in another L.A. hospital also had contracted a similar infection.[67] Within two weeks of that disclosure, the FDA responded with a comprehensive document addressing how to effectively "reprocess" complicated pieces of equipment that need to be completely sterilized between patients.[68] (Whoever said that the government cannot act quickly never met an agency afraid of lawsuits.)

About half a million patients each year have procedures involving this kind of device, and there have been numerous reports of infections from contaminated scopes, dating back to the 1980s.[69] Over the past two years, there were at least seventy-five reports of contaminated duodenoscopes, involving more than a hundred patients. But the last outbreak was different from the others, as it triggered a reaction from members of Congress who challenged the FDA to respond. The document that was prepared so quickly makes it clear that the FDA is being cautious about potential litigation. The report states: "FDA's guidance documents, including this guidance, do not establish legally enforceable responsibilities. Instead, guidances describe the Agency's current thinking on a topic and should be viewed only as recommendations." The purpose of the report is to recommend how to clean the devices, starting with a definition of cleaning ("physical removal of soil and contaminants") versus disinfection or sterilization (the process of killing all microorganisms). The components of duodenoscopes and other endoscopes are heat sensitive, so sterilization must be done by other approaches, such as chemical sterilization (hydrogen peroxide, ozone, and ethylene oxide can be used to kill microbes). The document also provides a guide to the resistance of microbes to germicidal chemicals, showing, for instance, that bacterial spores are most resistant and that vegetative bacteria and some viruses are less resistant.[70]

The point is that medical devices, while lifesavers, can also pose risks, and the FDA is unable to eliminate all risks. They can recommend and advise, but reprocessing for reuse, which involves cleaning and sterilizing these expensive pieces of equipment, is far from perfect. And it is not just endoscopes that can be problematic, as complications from medical devices can include those that are not reused, such as heart valves, coronary stents, artificial hips, pacemakers, and defibrillators, any of which can be defective or contaminated and lead to patient injuries and deaths. The FDA has the authority to recall products, but may be reluctant to do so if the device is necessary to save lives. The agency would have to carefully evaluate the risks versus the benefits of the device, taking into account how many cases have had complications, how serious or life threatening the diseases or injuries are, and how hazardous they might be in the future. Balancing risks and benefits drives many decisions in medical practice and can be very complicated.

We can legislate to improve our safety. Regulations and codes ensure individual and community health. Although the system of regulations and codes is not perfect, it protects us and helps monitor the products we are exposed to that can be hazardous and life threatening. We need to support government efforts to keep us safe, with the understanding that the agencies must remain independent entities. The agencies should not be influenced by corporations or others with interests that may conflict with public safety. Without government protections we will be at the mercy of the corporate profit motive, and that could be disastrous.

There are many solutions that will improve hand hygiene and health outcomes, ranging from the very personal decisions of whether or not to shake hands and how often to wash one's hands, to other strategies, such as employing emotions (disgust, shame, embarrassment), designing educational programs, reorganizing clinics with new SOPs, using technology, and government oversight. Each approach adds some measure of safety and the reassurance that we can keep pathogens at bay and live longer and healthier lives.

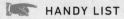 **HANDY LIST**

Top Ten Simple Solutions to Better Hand Hygiene

1   Don't shake hands, do the fist bump. If you do shake hands, be sure to wash up or use alcohol-based hand rub before touching your face or eating.

2   Keep your washing-up areas stocked with plenty of soap and clean cloth towels or paper towels. This is equally as important at home as it is at work.

3   Keep a bottle of alcohol-based hand rub handy, at work or on the road.

4   If you are a parent of small children, or a caretaker for a family member, keep your charge's hands clean.

5   Teach your children from the earliest ages to keep their hands clean, in particular, to wash after coming home from school, the playground, or other activities, and before eating.

6   If you are a supervisor at work, develop and encourage hygiene policies for your employees. Your initiative may be as modest or subtle as making sure there is soap and paper towels in the bathrooms and hand rub available in the office.

7   If you work in health care, be vigilant about hand hygiene, cooperate with hygiene policies, and take the initiative to be a role model for others.

8   If you are a patient, politely ask your healthcare worker to wash hands and don gloves. If you are advocating for a family member who is being treated, you should do the same. This is not the time to be bashful or worry about insulting someone.

9   If possible, when buying prepared food, be aware of how your food is handled and ask the food handler to wash hands or don gloves.

10 Learn about local health codes, and advocate for them. Encourage your legislators to develop policies, codes, and laws to further protect consumers.

The Future of Hand Hygiene
It's Not a Game

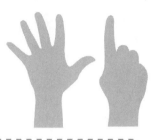

Apparently infectious diseases can be cool and fun, and that's why a board game called Pandemic has become popular among millennials. While many games are competitive and the goal is to prevail over your opponents, Pandemic is "a truly cooperative game where you all win or you all lose."[1] The game's website explains that "Four diseases have broken out in the world, and it is up to a team of specialists in various fields to find cures for these diseases before mankind is wiped out." Players take on different roles, such as medic, quarantine specialist, or scientist, and use strategies to cure and eradicate diseases before they spread throughout the world. The game board is a map of the world highlighting key cities in which epidemics can arise, such as New York, San Francisco, London, and Istanbul. When setting up the game, players place a research station in Atlanta, the actual home city of the Centers for Disease Control and Prevention (CDC). "Disease cubes" mark affected areas; and as cards are played, the number of "disease cubes" in particular cities grows, signaling the rapid rate of infections occurring within cities. If players do not treat diseases quickly enough, outbreaks occur, and all of the surrounding cities are affected.

This game is captivating to me, a professional germie, however, designing a game based on this theme may be trivializing the issue. Yet Pandemic is, after all, only a game; and to put it in perspective, Risk, one of the most popular board games of all time, was about world domination, and none of my friends who played it at the time wound up actually taking over any countries. In addition to serving as a way to fill a lazy afternoon with friends, perhaps games such as Pandemic will raise awareness of disease-related issues and get people thinking about hand hygiene. My daughter and son-in-law play Pandemic frequently with their friends; and as they play, they discuss the real-world implications of the issues, such as the importance of vaccinations.

If we can learn how to deal with infectious diseases on a day-to-day basis, when the threat is low, we will have a better chance of prevailing over infectious diseases when the risk is elevated during an outbreak of disease, or in the event of a bigger crisis of epidemic proportions or a global pandemic. But we need to prepare now. "Do you have what it takes to save humanity?" asks the Pandemic website. If all the players work together, cooperate, and think creatively, the answer is "yes."

Likewise, we can win the real game against infectious disease. In the developed world, in many respects we have made tremendous strides against contagion and infection. Through modern approaches to hygiene, antibiotics, and vaccination, as well as improved nutrition, the average life expectancy is almost double what it was a hundred years ago. Using vaccination programs, humanity won the war against smallpox, and practically eradicated polio and measles. However, success can breed complacency, and people who have never witnessed serious infectious diseases take the lives of their loved ones, or wipe out whole families, may not understand the importance of continued vigilance. Because of complacency we are beginning to lose some of the battles. The antivaccine movement is misleading people and attempting to convince them to reject vaccines that save lives. Drug-resistant bacteria arising in healthcare settings pose a threat to our health and safety. Lackadaisical approaches to hygiene can lead to spread of infectious diseases. And on the battlefront against infectious disease in developing countries, we have a long, long way to go. Fortunately, we still have many weapons in our arsenal against infectious diseases, and we are developing new strategies and approaches to understanding our complex relationship to microbes and the threat they may pose.

The Pandemic game has become so popular that there are now a number of expansion games, including Pandemic: On the Brink, Pandemic: Contagion, and my personal favorite, Pandemic: In the Lab. I have not actually played it yet, but I love the title. Pandemic: On the Brink comes with real petri dishes that are used to store and organize the "disease cubes," perhaps so that players can quarantine the diseases, until the next outbreak.

Is There Such a Thing as Too Clean?

One beautiful spring day when I was taking a walk and pushing my infant daughter in her stroller, I ran into a close friend. When my daughter began to cry, my friend popped her finger into my daughter's mouth to pacify her. I nearly had a stroke. My friend's intentions were benevolent, and she explained that she did the same with her own daughter because sucking a finger comforted her when she cried.

Clearly there are parents who have different approaches to hygiene when it comes to babies. A Swedish study reports that "Parental sucking of their infant's pacifier may reduce the risk of allergy development."[2] When my daughters' pacifiers fell on the floor, I always had a spare, so I could rinse off the dirty one later when clean water was available. But some resourceful parents will pick the pacifier off the floor and suck on it to cleanse it before popping it back in their infant's mouth, and apparently this idea is not as dreadful as it seems to me. The study underscores the complexity of our relationship with microorganisms, as it appears that exposing babies to certain microbes early in life may stimulate their immune systems, reducing the likelihood of developing allergies later on. The study compared 184 infants with regard to allergy development, focusing on several factors, including parental sucking of pacifiers, parental history of allergy, parental smoking, whether babies were born by Caesarean section or vaginally, whether they were breast-fed, the presence of a cat or dog at home, and parental level of education. Of all of those factors, only parental pacifier sucking and being born vaginally were significantly correlated with fewer allergies. The authors speculated that parental saliva exposed the babies to a set of microbes that stimulated their immune systems, leading to a lower incidence of asthma; reduced eczema and sensitization at eighteen months; and reduction in eczema at thirty-six months. Vaginal delivery also correlates with lower incidence of allergies, as the passage of the infant through the birth canal may expose her to vaginal microbes that appear to benefit the infant's immune system. Both vaginal delivery and parental pacifier sucking are individually associated with fewer allergies. And when tested, the microbes found in the mouths of babes who are exposed to parental saliva or born by vaginal delivery, or both, are different from those found in the mouths of other infants. On the other end of the spectrum, infants who were neither born vaginally nor exposed to parental saliva had the highest incidence of allergies, manifesting as eczema. This study supports the idea that beneficial microbes found in parental saliva and the vaginal canal can help infants to develop a healthy immune system. We still need to protect our children from the harmful microbes, and we do not want to take chances that they might pick up diseases from other people or from public places; but a certain set of microbes, generally from a healthy mother, helps to establish a healthy microbiome.

One more observation with regard to parental pacifier sucking is that saliva is no ordinary liquid; it is a complex mixture of biologically active materials. For instance, human saliva contains antibacterial substances, such as the enzyme lysozyme, which damages bacterial cell walls.[3] Canine (dog) saliva is likewise antimicrobial and has been shown to kill *E. coli* and *Streptococcus canis* bacteria, which explains why maternal grooming of pups with saliva is important to the newborns' health.[4] In addition, proteins called histatins, which are found in saliva, stimulate wound closing and facilitate healing, which may be why mouth lesions and cuts, continuously bathed in saliva, heal so much faster than skin lesions.[5] Histatins also have antifungal properties. So parental pacifier sucking may be beneficial to infants in several ways: by providing parental bacteria to stimulate the immune system; by providing antibacterial protection; and by providing histatins, which could protect the newborn's delicate oral tissues from lesions.

As we learned in chapter 1, the microbiome is a broad population of many types of microbes, most of which are harmless or even beneficial. It is good to expose babies to some microbes, but you still do not want your baby sucking on random shopping cart handles, pacifiers, or other objects. Dangerous germs are out there. The take-home lesson is that parental saliva is not necessarily going to harm the infant (unless the parent is sick) and may actually help her; and in addition, it appears that it is better for an infant to be born vaginally, if possible. The rate of Caesarian births has skyrocketed in the United States, and perhaps that can partially explain the recent dramatic increase in allergies. But that is the subject of a whole other book.

As we have shown, the native flora—bacteria of the skin and body— help to protect us from infections. Our skin and digestive systems are naturally colonized by benign strains of bacteria that help keep us healthy. When native species of bacteria are eliminated or reduced by using antibiotics or overwashing, pathogenic, disease-causing bacteria may move in, leading to illness. The overuse of cleansers, antimicrobial solutions, and antibiotics can be counterproductive. People with obsessive compulsive disorder (OCD) may overdo handwashing (and other behaviors), which can lead to skin disorders and other complications. The solution is finding a happy medium where cleanliness is achieved without destroying the delicate balance of native microbes found on and in the human body.

Microbiomes and Health

Science writer Michael Pollan wrote about microbiomes in a *New York Times Magazine* cover story. The cover, which pictures a huge golden Labrador licking a baby's face, provocatively promises an exposé on "The Secret Lives of Germs: What We Can Learn from Our Microbiome."[6] Pollan makes the point that our microbes are part and parcel of our bodies, and necessary for healthful functioning. He refers to himself as a "superorganism," a term that includes his own organs and tissues, plus several hundred species of microbes, the microbiome, which numbers around one hundred trillion cells. When we disrupt this population of microbes, for instance by taking antibiotics, it can have negative effects, leading to obesity, chronic diseases, and even some infections. "Some of my best friends are bacteria," declares Pollan.[7] In an interview, "Behind the Cover Story," Pollan expresses concerns about the Western microbiome and its lack of diversity, suggesting that perhaps we are too sterile. We need literally to play in the dirt, and to learn more about microbes in our diet, for instance those that ferment our food. "Exposure to soil is probably a good thing," he says. "Having a dog may be a good thing too."[8] The microbes that colonize our bodies naturally change over time and in response to drugs, diet, chemicals, and where we live. We each have a microbial fingerprint of sorts that can be left in traces on what we touch. The challenge will be to figure out what constitutes a healthy balance of microbes and how to achieve it. DNA technologies that are being used to map our genomes also will be helpful in mapping our individual microbiomes. And if the microbiome gets disrupted, perhaps we will know how to restore it to the proper balance.

The restoration of a balanced healthy microbiome is the goal of an experimental therapy called fecal transplantation. Patients with chronic gastrointestinal diseases, such as *C. difficile* infections that do not respond to other treatments, are candidates for this procedure. Healthy donors provide stool samples, or "fecal microbiota preparations," that are transferred into the patient's gut using an enema, a colonoscope, or a nasogastric tube. The donor's bacteria compete with the *C. difficile* and repopulate the intestine with healthy microbes. The future of this technique will rely on access to healthy microbiomes from stool donors. Healthy fecal matter is not as easy to obtain as one may think. A project called OpenBiome, which is a human stool bank, aims to maintain stocks of human feces so doctors will have ready access to the resource when fecal transplants become routine.[9]

The success of fecal transplant therapy will depend on researchers gaining a better understanding of which bacteria are helpful and which are harmful in the body. Genome sequencing of specific strains of bacteria can provide information on precisely what microbes are present. This process has become a valuable tool for diagnosis of infectious disease; and in the future, it could be applied to surveying entire microbiomes and developing approaches that are more sophisticated for restoring microbiomes than simply inserting random stool samples from someone else's gut.[10] A more individualized approach will be possible and is in line with the trend toward personalized medicine, that is, tailoring medical treatments to individuals.

Managing Microbes
Antibiotic Resistance

Antibiotics are prescribed for certain pathogenic bacterial infections, and they can be very effective in curing those infections. However, antibiotics are being misused and overprescribed, and there are complications that arise as a result of their overuse. Many doctors prescribe antibiotics for infections that have not been established to be bacterial and may well be viral in origin. This is counterproductive, as it does nothing to alleviate the infection, while it can destroy benign bacteria and encourage the growth of drug-resistant microbes.

While antibiotics save lives, they also disrupt the friendly bacteria and upset the delicate balance of microbes. The drugs typically target many types of bacteria, not just the ones that cause illness, so they can damage and destroy beneficial bacteria in humans, animals, and the environment. That is why oral antibiotics can lead to gastrointestinal problems such as diarrhea and nausea.

In addition to killing benign bacteria, another serious complication associated with the use of antibiotics is that combating bacteria with drugs can lead to the generation of antibiotic-resistant microbes. When an infected person or animal is treated with antibiotics, the infectious bacteria are killed. However, within the population of microbes there may be some mutants or variants that have the ability to evade or resist the drug; and when all the susceptible bacteria die, the drug-resistant ones can reemerge, become dominant, and flourish. That is why if a first round of antibiotics fails to cure an infection, the doctor may try a totally different drug, which may be effective in killing the resistant pathogens. But that second drug is not always successful, as multidrug-resistant bacteria can arise. When the disease-causing organisms cannot be defeated with conventional drugs, they become deadly dangers in clinical settings as they can spread from patient to patient, especially in weakened and immune-compromised patients, who may succumb to such a challenge. The medical profession is in danger of running out of options for treating multidrug-resistant bacteria.

Having noted this, since many microbes cause disease and death and need to be dealt with cautiously, antibiotics are useful. But there are first lines of defense that can reduce our exposure to microbes, and in turn reduce the need for antibiotics. Handwashing is one such strategy designed to reduce the risk of human disease, thereby reducing our need for antibiotics.

In agricultural settings antibiotics are used to treat sick animals, but they are also used prophylactically to prevent animals from contracting illnesses. Antibiotic treatments also are used to promote the growth of livestock, which is done from an economic motive not even related to the health of the animals. Since farming is big business, any approach that can squeeze additional profit from a product (such as growing bigger cows, pigs, or chickens) is often employed. But using antibiotics in this way increases the likelihood of generating antibiotic-resistant superbugs.

In September 2014 the President's Council of Advisors on Science and Technology (PCAST) prepared a report, "Combating Antibiotic Resistance," that offers a comprehensive approach to addressing the rise in antibiotic-resistant bacteria. A number of scientists and leaders from a wide spectrum of concerned agencies, institutions, and organizations were involved in the preparation of the report. Thomas Freiden, director of the Centers for Disease Control and Prevention; Francis Collins, director of the National Institutes of Health; Anthony Fauci, director of the National Institute of Allergy and Infectious Diseases; and Margaret Hamburg, commissioner of the Food and Drug Administration, were among the "experts consulted." The report clearly stated the problem: "PCAST identified several areas that require urgent attention and outlined a set of practical and actionable steps that the United States government should take over the next few years to bring the antibiotic-resistance crisis under control. Those steps focus on ways to improve our surveillance capabilities for resistant bacteria, increase the longevity of current antibiotics, and accelerate the rate at which new antibiotics and other interventions are discovered and developed."[11]

The PCAST report sets the stage for understanding the severity of the problem. The report recounts that at the turn of the twentieth century, as many as nine out of every thousand women died as a result of infections acquired from childbirth. At that time infant mortality rates soared in many cities, with up to 30 percent of children dying in their first year. People died from simple skin infections, pneumonia had a 30 percent mortality rate, and sore throats could lead to rheumatic fever and heart failure. Surgery was associated with high rates of infection and mortality. But antibiotics changed all that, providing a safe way to treat infections with few complications. However, because of the overuse of antibiotics we are jeopardizing the progress we have made, and this is threatening the recovery of patients. The report lists "current antibiotic-resistant threats in the United States," including some they classified as "urgent," for example, *Clostridium difficile*, which infects 250,000 per year, killing 14,000, and Carbapenem-Resistant Enterobacteriaceae (CRE), which infects 9,300 per year, with 610 deaths. Those categorized as "serious threats" include Methicillin-Resistant *Staphylococcus aureus* (MRSA, causing more than 80,000 infections, and more than 11,000 deaths per year), drug-resistant

Streptococcus pneumoniae (1.2 million cases, 7,000 deaths), and a host of others.[12]

The preparation of that report and its outcomes may be an example of government at its best. The PCAST report led to President Barack Obama's Executive Order of September 18, 2014, charging a task force with developing federal policies to combat antibiotic-resistant bacteria, as "a national security priority."[13] Six months later, the National Action Plan for Combating Antibiotic Resistant Bacteria was unveiled by the White House. The plan was outlined in a sixty-two-page document dated March 2015, with the main goals being to "slow the emergence of resistant bacteria and prevent spread of resistant infections," to support the development of diagnostic tests that will facilitate the identification of resistant bacteria, and to encourage and support research programs for developing new antibiotics and other approaches to combat infections. In addition, it proposes steps for developing collaborative programs with other world powers to prevent the global spread of these challenging superbugs and for conducting surveillance to keep those microbes in check.[14]

Many facets of the plan are to be implemented by 2020, including the reduction in incidence of MRSA and *C. difficile*. Major goals are to decrease the superfluous use of antibiotics in healthcare settings, reduce the use of antibiotics in livestock, and eliminate the indiscriminate use of antibiotics to promote growth in food animals. Some physicians prescribe antibiotics if there is only a chance an infection is bacterial. As mentioned previously, those drugs do not combat viral diseases. However, if fast, effective tests can be developed to discriminate between bacterial and viral infections, physicians may be able to limit the use of drugs to bacterial infections only. Reduced use of antibiotics will help to prevent the development and continued proliferation of resistant strains of bacteria. In order for all of this to be carried out, there will have to be cooperation of experts, organizations, and institutions in health care, agriculture, and drug manufacturing across the globe. Policies on the use of antibiotics in health care and agriculture will need to be developed, and regulations on the use of antibiotics in agriculture and the environment will have to be enforced. Just as in the board game, Pandemic, all the players will have to work together to save humanity.

The Global Problem

There are many places on our planet where people have rudimentary resources for hygiene. When there is not enough clean water and soap is a luxury item, hygiene issues seem insurmountable. However, it is possible, through international programs and cooperation, to assist and encourage the development of improved hygiene facilities in the least-developed areas of the globe. The WASH initiative works to provide adequate water, sanitation, and hygiene (acronym WASH) worldwide.[15] According to WHO and UNICEF data, two-and-a-half-billion people worldwide do not have access to an "improved sanitation facility,"[16] which is defined as "one that hygienically separates human excreta from human contact."[17] Human and animal waste are known to carry disease-causing germs, such as *Salmonella*, *E. coli*, and norovirus. In developed countries we take for granted that we have facilities for sanitary indoor defecation and waste disposal, but there are forty-five countries in the world where more than 50 percent of the people still do not use improved sanitation facilities, and open defecation is common. In the Western Hemisphere only Bolivia is in that most extreme category. Most countries in sub-Saharan Africa, India, Pakistan, Afghanistan, Nepal, Bhutan, Bangladesh, Cambodia, and Papua New Guinea round out the list of countries with dire hygienic conditions. The good news is that from 1990 to 2011 the open defecation rate declined from 24 to 15 percent worldwide; although in sub-Saharan Africa, the number of people defecating in the open is still increasing and now exceeds two hundred million people. Vietnam, Bangladesh, Peru, and Honduras experienced dramatic improvements in that period of time. For instance, Vietnam went from 40 percent open defecation to 3 percent, and Ethiopia went from 93 to 45 percent of the population with no improved sanitation facilities, which is a significant stride forward but still needs more progress.[18]

The world is moving in the right direction, but it still has a long way to go to provide the entire human population with sanitation facilities to maintain good health. Infectious disease can be transmitted by drinking contaminated water, exposure to contaminated water through washing or bathing, inadequate personal hygiene, and inadequate agricultural hygiene (i.e., fruits, vegetables, and meats contaminated with disease-causing microorganisms). A study analyzing WASH conditions—that is, water, sanitation, and hygiene as related to infectious disease in 145 countries—revealed that in 2012 more than half a million diarrhea deaths were attributable to inadequate drinking water, and an additional 280,000 to inadequate sanitation. In this statistical analysis of world data, the authors estimated the number of people who died because of inadequate hand hygiene at 297,000 individuals.[19] This study also estimated that 361,000 deaths in children age five and under could have been prevented by better access to safe water, sanitation, and hygiene. The authors conclude that "reliable piped water, community sewage with treatment, and hand hygiene" are necessary to reduce the risk of infection in those populations.[20] For lack of clean water, basic latrines, and routine handwashing, hundreds of thousands of human lives were lost.

There are organizations working to remedy global hygiene issues. One example is the Global Public-Private Partnership for Handwashing (PPPHW), which is a coalition of groups, including major private corporations with commercial interests in hygiene, academic institutions (the State University of New York at Buffalo, and the London School of Hygiene and Tropical Medicine), as well as the organization FHI360. FHI360 (formerly Family Health International) is a North Carolina–based organization with offices in New York City, Boston, Washington, D.C., Bangkok, Thailand, and Pretoria, South Africa. That organization, whose goal it is to improve lives, human development, and human potential, received more than $600 million in grants from the U.S. government in 2013 alone (from the National Institutes of Health, the CDC, Department of State, Department of Education, and Department of Health and Human Services), as well as millions of dollars in private donations, so they have significant resources to make a difference in global hygiene.[21]

The PPPHW includes three huge corporations in their coalition of international stakeholders. The three multinational manufacturers of handwashing products, Colgate-Palmolive, Unilever, and Proctor & Gamble, are business competitors, but they came together for a common cause, to contribute to the programs of the PPPHW. Colgate-Palmolive, one of the founding members of the PPPHW, manufactures Irish Spring soap, Softsoap liquid hand soap, and various types of body wash. "A cleaner, healthy environment is important to Colgate not only because it's the right thing to do, but also because it makes good business sense. . . . Colgate aims to provide handwashing awareness to over 50 million households."[22] Unilever's homepage shows a photo of an Indian woman with three small children, and the slogan, "Brands with a purpose." The website boldly claims that their products are "brands used by two billion people every day." They produce Dove and Lux soaps and their more than one-hundred-year-old brand Lifebuoy, whose distinctive red soap bar is claimed to provide "improved hygiene protection."[23] Proctor & Gamble makes many household cleaning products, such as Tide laundry detergent, Bounty paper towels, Crest toothpaste, Safeguard soap, and the classic Ivory soap. The webpage for Ivory declares, "This isn't your grandmother's soap. This is your great-great grandmother's soap . . . If it's good enough for your Nana, it's good enough for you."[24]

The mission of the PPPHW is to bring together "the expertise, experience, ideas, resources and reach of the public and private sectors around the world to promote handwashing with soap." They explain that handwashing with soap is a "'do-it-yourself vaccine' that prevents infections and saves lives."[25] In that spirit, on October 15, 2008, the PPPHW launched Global Handwashing Day as part of the United Nations International Year of Sanitation; and every year since then October 15 is designated Global Handwashing Day, a day committed to handwashing-related programs and activities. One such program on "Exploring New Ideas in Hygiene Integration, Innovations and Insights into Behavioral Drivers" was held in Washington, D.C., on October 15, 2014.[26]

Dr. Timothy Mastrow, the secretariat of FHI360, opened that event by observing that the Ebola epidemic raging in western Africa heightens world awareness of how inadequate levels of hygiene can be a threat to all humanity. Dr. Tina Sanghvi discussed a successful initiative with regard to handwashing, the "Alive and Thrive" program in Bangladesh. In many Bangladeshi families, mothers exclusively breastfeed their infants for six months. But when complementary feeding is introduced, the incidence of infant infection soars as the foods introduced into their diet are highly contaminated because of poor handwashing and hygiene practices. In those communities handwashing is not part of the social norms, and there is little appreciation of its benefits. In addition, many homes are not set up with or convenient to handwashing facilities, so it is bothersome to wash hands before feeding the baby. By using educational materials and visual aids, the Alive and Thrive program reached many mothers, and in a short period of time handwashing before feeding increased from about 3 to 5 percent of mothers to 58 percent.[27]

Other speakers at the PPPHW program discussed innovative handwashing stations that were invented and are being promoted for street vendors in India, where street food is an integral part of the culture but hygiene is lacking. The "Tippy Tap" is a hands-free device that can be used almost anywhere to hygienically wash hands, using as little as 40 ml (about $1\frac{1}{3}$ ounces) of water per washing. The Tippy Tap is simply a large plastic jug full of clean water, with a small hole punched near the top. The jug is hung from its handle on a horizontal stick, and by pulling a rope (or stepping on a foot lever attached to a rope) the jug tilts and releases a small stream of water. The clean water stream is used to wet the hands. Soap on a rope is hung nearby to lather up, and then the hands are rinsed with clean water from the Tippy Tap. Customers of the street vendors are encouraged to preferentially patronize vendors who wash hands, thereby making it profitable for the vender to incorporate handwashing into a successful street vendor business model.[28]

Another smaller company involved in charitable work is named Soap-Box Soaps. As their name implies, SoapBox Soaps is a "for-purpose company" with a social mission. Founded five years ago by a group of young entrepreneurs, the name SoapBox conjures up an old-time rabble-rouser with a cause, standing on his soapbox on a street corner, proclaiming his opinions to the gathering crowd. At the PPPHW program, SoapBox's director of communications Cici Pandol explained how they achieve their social mission. Since SoapBox wants to make a global impact, she explained, "For every bar of soap you buy, we give a bar of soap." They accomplish this by collecting used hotel soap bar remnants, sanitizing them, and re-forming them into new bars. Seventy percent are given to homeless shelters and food banks in the United States.[29] The rest are donated internationally to relief efforts around the world. Most recently they donated to emergency relief in Nepal after the 2015 earthquake.[30] Their "buy one, give one" product policy extends to other products they sell as well. For every bottle of liquid soap sold, they donate a one-month supply of clean water. For every bottle of body wash, they donate a year's supply of vitamins. They sum up their philosophy with the catchy phrase, "Soap = hope. That's our plan, really. Use soap to improve the world."[31]

Immigration and Infections

We now live in a global society, which gives us the responsibility to help developing nations; this is vital not only for humanitarian reasons, but for selfish ones as well. Germs know no borders; humans carry microbes wherever they go, and people travel worldwide to places where there are common as well as less familiar deadly diseases.

During the nineteenth and twentieth centuries, immigration to the United States involved medical screening at ports of entry. At Ellis Island, where from 1892 to 1954 more than twelve million immigrants were processed, the staff of U.S. Public Health Service physicians conducted cursory medical inspections of hundreds of thousands of people each year in order to cull immigrants who might be a burden to society because of illness or disability. They paid special attention to screening out people with contagious diseases, such as trachoma, an infectious disease of the eye that, if untreated, caused blindness in three out of four of its victims. The screening for trachoma was a ghastly affair, and frequently involved the use of an unsanitized buttonhook to evert the eyelid and reveal the infection.[32]

Today almost anyone can enter the United States, regardless of disease or disability. However, in October 2014, after Thomas Eric Duncan succumbed to Ebola on U.S. soil, President Obama and the Centers for Disease Control and Prevention ordered all travelers from the Ebola hotspots Sierra Leone, Guinea, and Liberia to be screened. A CDC fact sheet, updated in March 2015, explains "how we can prevent the spread of Ebola in the United States by screening travelers at airports, controlling their movement and monitoring their activities."[33]

As of this writing, the first stage of screening occurs as travelers leave the three countries stricken with the epidemic. The exit screening steps include checking the temperature of travelers and asking questions about their health and possible exposure to Ebola. At this time there are no direct flights from Sierra Leone, Guinea, or Liberia to the United States, so travelers pass through other countries on the way and are subject to whatever restrictions the other countries impose. Those who continue on to the

United States are required to arrive at one of five international airports: New York's JFK Airport, Newark's Liberty International Airport, Washington Dulles, Chicago O'Hare, or Hartsfield-Jackson Atlanta International Airport. In the airport the travelers go through a process called entry screening. The Department of Homeland Security staff ask the travelers questions concerning possible exposure to Ebola, take their temperatures, and check for any other disease symptoms. They also obtain contact information for each traveler. Each person is given a Check and Report Ebola (CARE) Kit, which contains an informational booklet and health log, a digital thermometer, a prepaid twenty-one-day cell phone, and a CDC CARE card. The booklet instructs each traveler on how to take their temperature twice a day and how to enter the information on temperature and symptoms into the log. If any symptoms of Ebola appear (for instance, stomach pain, vomiting, diarrhea, muscle pain, etc.) and/or if their temperature exceeds 100.4 degrees F. (38 degrees C.), they are instructed to not go out in public and to get care immediately by calling the local health department (listed in the booklet). The CDC CARE card is required to be carried at all times, as it identifies the individual as someone who has "recently returned from a country with an Ebola outbreak."[34]

This approach to screening individuals for deadly diseases upon entry into the United States is a positive step in the strategy to keep the U.S. population safe, and it is well intentioned. However, it requires the cooperation of people who may have been exposed abroad, and it relies on monitoring and reporting to the appropriate authorities. Not everyone wants to be under the scrutiny of authorities or is conscientious about taking temperature and recording data. There are real and substantial risks from germs that reside in our country, as well as germs from abroad. So once again, a prudent approach to lowering your risk of disease is to . . . you guessed it . . . wash your hands.

A Song of Handwashing

Dr. Layla McCay, secretariat director of PPPHW, wrapped up the PPPHW event noting, "There are still millions of children dying because of diseases that can be prevented by handwashing." But there is progress and hope for better hygiene and better health in the future, and she ended the program by playing a video of a recently released song by the Nigerian singer, Sunny Neji, who uses a catchy tune to deliver the important message, "Wash Your Hands O!":[35]

Wash your hands O! Wash your hands O!
Wash your hands before you cook, wash your hands before you eat,
Wash your hands before you serve food, wash your hands O.
If you go toilet or change pickin diaper, wash your hands O.
If you touch sick person or touch animals, wash your hands O.
Dirty hands dey carry disease O. Wey dey make plenty people sick.
Everyday children dem dey die O, From habit wey we fit to stop.
Prevention is cheaper than cure; Hospital na plenty money.
Wash your hands with soap and water, wash your hands O.
Prevent Ebola, prevent diarrhea, wash your hands O.
Prevent cholera, prevent pneumonia, wash your hands O.
Prevent typhoid and other infections, wash your hands O.
So tell your son and tell your daughter! Wash your hands O.
I say tell your father and tell your mother, wash your hands O.
Handwashing saves lives!

This catchy song shows that entertainment can be used to encourage handwashing, in a pleasant, positive way.

Other ways to encourage handwashing include the two "Hygiene Holidays" that are listed on www.cute-calendar.com.[36] In addition to Global Handwashing Day, which is observed on October 15 (discussed previously), the World Health Organization (WHO), in partnership with the CDC and other organizations, designated May 5 as World Hand Hygiene Day. Every year the WHO chooses a theme for the day. The theme in 2015 was the importance of handwashing in preventing the spread of antimicrobial-resistant diseases.[37] Organizations around the world schedule events in honor of the May 5 observance. Clearly, hand hygiene is so essential that it deserves two holidays, in May and October.

Brainstorming for the Future

The problem of inadequate hand hygiene continues to vex us. Improved behavior and solutions can come about only by educating adults as well as children, changing attitudes about hygiene, and working together within the context of a diversity of beliefs and cultures. To succeed, adults will need to relearn the practice of hand hygiene they learned as tots and pledge to practice it consistently, even when Mom is no longer in the picture. In hospital settings healthcare professionals will have to be vigilant about hand hygiene and the proper use of gloves, and patients will have to insist that doctors and nurses wash their hands before touching them.

Society has changed dramatically with regard to what behavior is acceptable and what is rejected. In the same way that many nonsmokers protest when a smoker violates "no smoking" rules in a public space, expectations and peer pressure will lead to consistent handwashing, and nonwashers will be shunned. Initially, patients may feel awkward enforcing those principles, but it will become part of the culture and expected of all healthcare workers without exception, so no one, except the violators, will feel singled out or offended.

New products will be developed to manage microbes, including new antibiotics, as recommended by the president's National Action Plan for Combating Antibiotic-Resistant Bacteria. Antibiotics will be used more judiciously, reducing the incidence of drug-resistant forms. Other types of antimicrobials will be developed to use in concert with alcohol-based hand rubs and soap and water. Perhaps we can learn a thing or two from nature and take advantage of antimicrobial body chemistry. Our tears, saliva, mucous, and even ear wax have antimicrobial properties. If we can adapt the chemistry of bodily secretions, new products may be available that could pose little risk, with enormous benefit.

When a pandemic arises, there is a temptation to panic, but the best course of action is to use all the tools of science and medicine we can muster to fight it. This was done effectively in Liberia, one of the three countries that were Ebola hotspots from 2014 to 2015. On May 9, 2015, after an estimated 4,700 deaths from the disease, including hundreds of healthcare workers, Liberia was declared by the World Health Organization to be free from Ebola.[38] At the start of the crisis, healthcare workers in Liberia had no protective suits, and hospitals lacked basic amenities, such as running water, electricity, and gloves. The inadequate healthcare system made it impossible to properly respond, and the disease spiraled out of control.[39] The victory was possible because healthcare resources from all over the world were used judiciously to turn a desperate situation into a deliberate, organized approach to managing the disease. Some of the solutions included providing clean water and power for clinics, ensuring that gloves and protective suits were available for healthcare workers, isolating afflicted people, handling remains of victims appropriately, and disposing of medical wastes properly. It was a victory for medical science and hygiene.

Practical Guidelines

This book has provided many tips and much advice designed to encourage handwashing to reduce the risk of infection and improve health. From a practical perspective it is possible to adopt simple behaviors that will make a difference. The most important advice I can offer is that children should be taught the importance of hand hygiene from very early on, and those lessons should be reinforced as they grow up. It is necessary to provide the tools of good hygiene and guide and encourage good hygiene habits to successfully pass on those important lessons. Providing individual towels for each child, along with accessible soap and clean water, and consistently enforcing the rules of handwashing after the toilet and before meals are major steps in making hand hygiene the expected behavior, and a routine part of life.

If you are aware of germs and high-risk behaviors related to microbes, when there is infectious disease (even a cold) in the household, you may be able to keep it from spreading. Dispose of dirty tissues right away, do not share personal items such as utensils, cups, towels, or toys from a sick child or adult, and keep the sick family member as far away from others as is practical. It may seem difficult, but it is worth it, as it reduces the chances of spreading the disease throughout the household.

From a broader perspective, there are policies and trends that have changed our microbial environment, leading to disruptions of our personal microbiomes as well as the microbes around us. For instance, in the United States there is a high incidence of induced births, and induction of labor is associated with an elevated risk of Caesarian births. It is now known that children born by Caesarian section have different microbiomes from those born vaginally, and a higher incidence of allergies, eczema, and asthma. So entering the world via the birth canal frequently confers a health advantage to the newborn.

Antibiotic-resistant bacteria are serious threats to humanity. This is not an American or partisan or religious issue; it is a global issue. And if our arsenal of drugs becomes impotent, fighting antibiotic-resistant bacteria may be a war that we are all in danger of losing. We need to make research on antibiotic resistance and development of new antibiotics a worldwide priority.

Patients must be assertive about hand hygiene, and medical professionals need to be more vigilant. Proper handwashing in clinical settings saves lives. In the same vein, while handshaking is a courteous gesture, it is not necessary and can be hazardous in medical environments. A friendly nod and a smile can replace a handshake, and while a smile can spread goodwill, it does not spread germs. In addition, neckties are simply unnecessary in the healthcare setting. Our society is getting more casual with regard to dress codes, so why not abolish neckties in hospitals? If you must wear a tie, make it a bow tie—at least it will not dangle and thus is less likely to pick up germs.

In theory, warm-air dryers and jet-air dryers seem like good ideas. In practice, even if you do have the patience to get your hands dry with these devices, there is evidence that they blow germs into the environment and spray and broadcast them great distances as aerosols and onto surfaces. And if you do not have the patience for air dryers, you walk away with wet hands, which are more likely to pick up and spread germs. Get rid of air hand dryers in public restrooms, and provide paper towels instead.

Scientists are making outstanding progress in discovering how genes work, and that will give us unprecedented power to understand disease-causing organisms. We need to commit government resources for research on microbes and microbiomes. Who would imagine some of the technological advances we have witnessed in our lifetimes? I am not talking about an octogenarian's lifetime or even my own. I am talking to generation X and millennials. In the past twenty to thirty years we have witnessed outstanding developments that change the way we live our lives. These developments include remarkable inventions that are used by ordinary people: The Internet, the smart phone (a combined computer, picture phone, video camera, music collection, library, and encyclopedia of all world knowledge in your pocket), the electric car, solar power, not to mention the sequenced human genome, reproductive and genetic technology, and artificial joints, lenses, limbs, and organs, which many of you will need in your lifetimes. We must support research on microorganisms, as we need to stay at least one step ahead of disease-causing germs. The technology is available, and the biological tools will enable us to develop a healthier environment and world.

Education about hygiene on the local and global levels will help keep us healthy and improve conditions worldwide. Small innovations, such as the Tippy Tap portable sink and washing with soap and water, save lives. Working worldwide on improving sanitation and hygiene will raise the quality of life for millions of people.

Finally, do your part. In the words of Sunny Neji, "Wash your hands O . . . Wash your hands before you cook. Wash your hands before you eat . . . I say tell your son and tell your daughter! Wash your hands O . . . Handwashing saves lives!"[40]

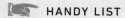 **HANDY LIST**

Keeping Kids Healthy:
How to Reduce Risk of Infection in the Home

1 Provide separate designated hand and bath towels for each child—on a separate towel ring or rod—and launder them regularly.
2 Provide soap that is easy to reach and use.
3 Monitor handwashing in very young children.
4 Consistently insist that children wash hands after various activities and before eating.
5 Minimize sharing of cups, utensils, and so on, among children.
6 Disinfect the toys of sick children before sharing.
7 Teach children proper use and disposal of facial tissues for sneezes and blowing nose.
8 Use clean bedding for each person; for sleepovers provide a bed with clean bedding.
9 Hold children's hands on a regular basis to keep them safe and communicate your love.

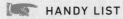 **HANDY LIST**

Take-Home Lessons:
How to Survive the Global Germ Age

1   Be born vaginally—it's a good start on establishing your microbiome. Oh, yeah, and ask your mother to suck your pacifier. (Seriously though, the obstetrics medical community should make a commitment to encourage and support vaginal deliveries and reduce the incidence of Caesarians.)

2   Combat antibiotic-resistant bacteria; develop policies and restrictions on the needless use of antibiotics. Use antibiotics sparingly, only when absolutely necessary. Develop new antibiotics that work via different mechanisms to inhibit and kill bacteria.

3   Empower patients; insist on handwashing by healthcare professionals.

4   Abolish and avoid handshaking in healthcare facilities. Try a friendly nod and a smile instead.

5   Ban neckties in healthcare facilities.

6   Remove hand blowers from all public restrooms and provide paper towels.

7   Commit funds to support research on microbes, microbiomes, and the implementation of the National Action Plan for Combating Antibiotic-Resistant Bacteria.

8   Establish and enforce rigorous policies and regulations for sanitizing airplanes, cruise ships, and other public places.

9   Purell and other alcohol-based hand rubs really work. Keep them close at hand.

10 Do whatever is needed to encourage hand hygiene. Start with education, entertainment, rewards, and pride. Use shame and disgust if necessary.

11 Support international efforts to improve water, sanitation, and hygiene worldwide.

12 Wash your hands at appropriate times.

Epilogue
I Want to Hold Your Hand

When babies are born, we admire and count their ten little fingers and ten little toes. The small hand's grasp reflex appears at birth, and the image of a tiny newborn hand grabbing his mommy's or daddy's finger, and bonding in a special way, is precious and moving. We laugh when our babies discover their hands, waving them in front of their own faces. We teach them hand gestures, such as how to clap and wave "bye-bye." We play hand games like patty-cake, we touch and tickle them, showing them our love, and teaching them about the world. As they grow, we hold our children's hands to keep them safe while crossing the street and to keep them close by.

"I Want to Hold Your Hand" was the Beatles' first American number one song on the Billboard Hot 100 Chart in 1964, and in 2013 it was ranked the Billboard forty-fourth biggest hit of all time. It was a song with a simple message that touched everyone, as holding hands is a universal expression of love. I have fond memories of holding my mother's hand as she guided me on ice skates on our tiny neighborhood pond. I held my best friend's hand when we were old enough to ice skate together without a grown-up. I held my boyfriend's hand when we skated together for the first time; now we are grandparents together, and we still hold hands.

When my mother was in the intensive care unit, I frequently held her hands, wiped them clean, and clipped her nails when needed. When my father was in the advanced stages of Parkinson's disease, we were fortunate to have caretakers who kept him comfortable and attended to his many needs. But there were times when I washed his hands and clipped his fingernails, and he appreciated this simple act that he himself could no longer manage. These quiet moments together were memories I cherish. When my father was rushed to the hospital on his last day of life, I accompanied him in the ambulance, holding his hand all the way. In the emergency room, I stayed with him; and before he was wheeled away to be sedated and intubated, I squeezed his hand and told him "I love you." My mother's last moments were with me in the hospital room, and I held her hand as she passed from this world.

For most of us, our hands are with us from before we are born to when we leave this life. We use them to touch and feel, to explore, carry, create, write, gesture, applaud, and greet. Our twenty-first century hands type and text and tweet. Keep your hands clean to keep yourself healthy. Be a hand-hygiene role model, and make the world a safer place, one pair of hands at a time.

NOTES

Preface: Hands Can Be Hazardous to Your Health

1. Miryam Z. Wahrman, Susan E. Gagnier, Diane R. Kobrin, Paul J. Higgins, and Leonard H. Augenlicht, "Cellular and Molecular Changes in 3T3 Cells Transformed Spontaneously or by DNA Transfection," *Tumor Biology* 6 (1985): 41–56.

2. Miryam Z. Wahrman, Leonard H. Augenlicht, and Paul J. Higgins, "Alterations in Growth Properties and Cellular Proteins of Cloned Hamster Lung Fibroblasts during Long-Term Culture," *Oncology* 41 (1984): 49–54.

3. Leonard H. Augenlicht, Miryam Z. Wahrman, Heidi Halsey, Leigh Anderson, John Taylor, and Martin Lipkin, "Expression of Cloned Sequences in Biopsies of Human Colonic Tissue and in Colonic Carcinoma Cells Induced to Differentiate *In Vitro*," *Cancer Research* 47 (1987): 6017–21.

4. P. J. Higgins, E. Borenfreund, M. Z. Wahrman, and A. Bendich, "*In Vitro* Consequences of Sperm-Somatic Cell Interactions," *European Journal of Cancer* 16 (1980): 1047–55.

5. M. Wahrman, J. Reyniak, A. Dunaif, D. Sperling, and J. Gordon, "Human Egg Pathology: Oocyte Recovery, and Egg Morphology as Related to Patient Diagnosis, Fertilization Rate and Early Development," *J. Gynaec. Endocrin.* 1 (1985): 12–19.

6. Patricia E. Barg, Miryam Z. Wahrman, Beth E. Talansky, and Jon W. Gordon, "Capacitated, Acrosome Reacted but Immotile Sperm, When Microinjected under the Mouse Zona Pellucida, Will Not Fertilize the Oocyte," *Journal of Experimental Zoology* 237 (1986): 365–74.

7. M. Z. Wahrman, J. R. Voos, R. H. Chesney, J. M. Werth, and E. E. Gardner, "Biotechnology at William Paterson College: Educating Students for the Genetics Revolution," in *The Genetics Revolution* (Washington, DC: Community College Press, 1998), 122–25.

8. Mukesh K. Sahni, Stamatios Spanos, Miryam Z. Wahrman, and Gurdial M. Sharma, "Marine Corrinoid-Binding Proteins for the Direct Determination of Vitamin B$_{12}$ by Radioassay," *Analytical Biochemistry* 289 (2001): 68–76.

9. M. K. Sahni, M. Z. Wahrman, V. Belenky, and G. M. Sharma, "Secondary Metabolites of Marine Organisms," in *New Developments in Marine Biotechnology*, ed. Y. Le Gal and H. O. Halvorson (New York: Plenum, 1998), 41–47.

10. Miryam Z. Wahrman and Sutian Zhu, "Haploid and Diploid Cell Cultures from a Haplo-Diploid Insect," *Invertebrate Reproduction and Development* 24 (1993): 79–86.

11. Jaishri Menon and Miryam Z. Wahrman, "Differential Response of Tail and

Body Epidermis of *Rana catesbeiana* Tadpoles *In Vitro* to Cisplatin," *In Vitro: Cellular and Developmental Biology (Animal)* 35 (1999): 8–11. Jaishri Menon and Miryam Z. Wahrman, "Ultrastructural Observations on Effects of Different Concentrations of Calcium and Thyroxine *In Vitro* on Larval Epidermal Cells of *Rana Catesbeiana* Tadpoles," *In Vitro: Cellular and Developmental Biology (Animal)* 37 (2001): 283–92.

12. Miryam Z. Wahrman, "Bioethics," in *Encyclopedia of Social Problems*, ed. Vincent Parrillo (Thousand Oaks, CA: Sage, 2008), 78–80. Miryam Z. Wahrman, "Fruit of the Womb: Artificial Reproductive Technologies and Jewish Law," *Journal of Gender, Race and Justice (University of Iowa College of Law)* 9 (2005): 109–36.

13. Miryam Z. Wahrman, *Brave New Judaism: When Science and Scripture Collide* (Hanover, NH: University Press of New England / Brandeis University Press, 2002; paperback edition, 2004).

14. Dror Cantrell, Oded Shamriz, Matan J. Cohen, Zvi Stern, Colin Block, and Mayer Brezis, "Hand Hygiene Compliance by Physicians: Marked Heterogeneity due to Local Culture?" *American Journal of Infection Control* 37 (2009): 301–5.

15. A. P. Jepson, C. McDougall, A. Clark, A. Bateman, G. Williamson, and M. E. Kaufmann, "Finger Rings Should Be Removed Prior to Scrubbing," *Journal of Hospital Infection* 64 (2006): 197–98.

16. Ibid.

17. Ibid.

18. Pennsylvania Food Code (Title 7, Chapter 46.136).

19. Theodore W. Pope, Peter T. Ender, William K. Woelk, Michael Koroscil, and Thomas Koroscil, "Bacterial Contamination of Paper Currency," *Southern Medical Journal* 95 (2002): 1408–10.

1. Handwashing Habits, Hygiene, and Health

1. Food and Drug Administration, *Retail Food Protection: Employee Health and Personal Hygiene Handbook*. Publication no. IFS 04. (Adapted from the FDA 2005 Food Code.) http://www.fda.gov/Food/GuidanceRegulation/RetailFoodProtection/IndustryandRegulatoryAssistanceandTrainingResources/ucm113827.htm.

2. Frederick Soddy, *Science and Life: Aberdeen Addresses* (New York: Dutton, 1920), 7–8.

3. Nicholas A. Eisele, Thomas Ruby, Amanda Jacobson, Paolo S. Manzanillo, Jeffery S. Cox, Lilian Lam, Lata Mukundan, Ajay Chawla, and Denise Monack, "Salmonella Require the Fatty Acid Regulator PPARδ for the Establishment of a Metabolic Environment Essential for Long-Term Persistence," *Cell Host and Microbe* 14 (2013): 171–82.

4. Donald G. McNeil Jr., "Bacteria Study Offers Clues to Typhoid Mary Mystery," *New York Times*, August 27, 2013.

5. Ted R. Johnson and Christine L. Case, *Laboratory Experiments in Microbiology*, 7th ed. (San Francisco: Pearson Education, 2004), chaps. 24, 26, and 46.

6. P. M. Donaldson, B. Naylor, J. W. Lowe, and D. R. Gouldesbrough, "Rapidly Fatal Necrotizing Fasciitis Caused by *Streptococcus pyogenes*," *Journal of Clinical Pathology* 46 (1993): 617–20.

7. Hampton Sides, "To Survive Flesh-Eating Bacteria," *Reader's Digest*, July 2014, 122–23.

8. Elizabeth A. Grice, Heidi H. Kong, Sean Conlan, Clayton B. Deming, Joie Davis, Alice C. Young, NISC Comparative Sequencing Program, Gerard G. Bouffard, Robert W. Blakesley, Patrick R. Murray, Eric D. Green, Maria L. Turner, and Julia A. Segre, "Topographical and Temporal Diversity of the Human Skin Microbiome," *Science* 324 (2009): 1190–92.

9. Donald G. McNeil, "Four Germs Cause Most of Infants' Severe Diarrhea," *New York Times*, May 21, 2013.

10. Kelly A. Reynolds, Pamela M. Watt, Stephanie A. Boone, and Charles P. Gerba, "Occurrence of Bacteria and Biochemical Markers on Public Surfaces," *International Journal of Environmental Health Research* 15 (2005): 225–34.

11. Krissi M. Hewitt, Charles P. Gerba, Sheri L. Maxwell, and Scott T. Kelley, "Office Space Bacterial Abundance and Diversity in Three Metropolitan Areas," PLOS ONE 7, no. 5 (2012): e37849, doi:10.1371/journal.pone.0037849.

12. Peter Andrey Smith, "Mapping the Great Indoors," *New York Times*, May 27, 2013.

13. Jiri Hulcr, Andrew M. Latimer, Jessica B. Henley, Nina R. Rountree, Noah Fierer, Andrea Lucky, Margaret D. Lowman, and Robert R. Dunn. "A Jungle in There: Bacteria in Belly Buttons Are Highly Diverse, but Predictable." *PLOS ONE* 7, no. 11 (2012): e47712, doi:10.1371/journal.pone.0047712.

14. Ibid.

15. Robert R. Dunn, Noah Fierer, Jessica B. Henley, Jonathan W. Leff, and Holly L. Menninger, "Home Life: Factors Structuring the Bacterial Diversity Found within and between Homes." *PLOS ONE* 8, no. 5 (2013): e64133, doi:10.1371/journal.pone.0064133.

16. Ibid.

17. Ibid.

18. Scott T. Kelley and Jack A. Gilbert, "Studying the Microbiology of the Indoor Environment," *Genome Biology* 14 (2013): 202, doi:10.1186/gb-2013-14-2-202.

19. Ibid.

20. Ibid.

21. Ibid.

22. Ebrahim Afshinnekoo, Cem Meydan, Shanin Chowdhury, Dyala Jaroudi, Collin Boyer, Nick Bernstein, Julia M. Maritz, Darryl Reeves, Jorge Gandara, Sagar

Chhangawala, Sofia Ahsanuddin, Amber Simmons, Timothy Nessel, Bharathi Sundaresh, Elizabeth Pereira, Ellen Jorgensen, Sergios-Orestis Kolokotronis, Nell Kirchberger, Isaac Garcia, David Gandara, Sean Dhanraj, Tanzina Nawrin, Yogesh Saletore, Noah Alexander, Priyanka Vijay, Elizabeth M. Henaff, Paul Zumbo, Michael Walsh, Gregory D. O'Mullan, Scott Tighe, Joel T. Dudley, Anya Dunaif, Sean Ennis, Eoghan O'Halloran, Tiago R. Magalhaes, Braden Boone, Angela L. Jones, Theodore R. Muth, Katie Schneider Paolantonio, Elizabeth Alter, Eric E. Shadt, Jeanne Garbarino, Robert J. Prill, Jane M. Carlton, Shawn Levy, and Christopher E. Mason, "Geospatial Resolution of Human and Bacterial Diversity with City-Scale Metagenomics," *Cell Systems* (2015): 1–15. http://dx.doi.org/10.1016/j.cels.2015.01 .001.

23. Ibid.

24. Ibid.

25. Ibid.

26. Ibid.

27. http://retractionwatch.com/2015/07/31/plague-or-anthrax-on-the-subway -think-again-says-now-corrected-study/.

28. Afshinnekoo et al., "Geospatial Resolution of Human and Bacterial Diversity."

29. http://retractionwatch.com/the-center-for-scientific-integrity/.

30. Afshinnekoo et al., "Geospatial Resolution of Human and Bacterial Diversity."

31. Ibid.

32. Tiago R. Magalhães, Jillian P. Casey, Judith Conroy, Regina Regan, Darren J. Fitzpatrick, Naisha Shah, Joao Sobral, and Sean Ennis, "HGDP and HapMap Analysis by Ancestry Mapper Reveals Local and Global Population Relationships," *PLOS ONE* 7 (2012): e49438. doi:10.1371/journal.pone.0049438.

33. Afshinnekoo et al., "Geospatial Resolution of Human and Bacterial Diversity."

34. Ibid.

35. Daniel Smith, John Alverdy, Gary An, Maureen Coleman, Sylvia Garcia-Houchins, Jessica Green, Kevin Keegan, Scott T. Kelley, Benjamin C. Kirkup, Larry Kociolek, Hal Levin, Emily Landon, Paula Olsiewski, Rob Knight, Jeffrey Siegel, Stephen Weber, and Jack Gilbert. "The Hospital Microbiome Project: Meeting Report for the 1st Hospital Microbiome Project Workshop on Sampling Design and Building Science Measurements, Chicago, USA, June 7–8, 2012," *Standards in Genomic Sciences* 8 (2013): 112–17.

36. Ibid.

37. Carrie Arnond, "Rethinking Sterile: The Hospital Microbiome," *Environmental Health Perspectives* 122 (2014): A182–A187.

38. Ibid.

39. Noah Fierer, Micah Hamady, Christian L. Lauber, and Rob Knight, "The Influence of Sex, Handedness, and Washing on the Diversity of Hand Surface Bacteria," *Proceedings of the National Academy of Sciences* 105 (2008): 17994–99.

40. Ibid.

41. Ibid.

42. Ibid.

43. Marilyn Chase, "Hand Washers Rise, but to Only 78%," *Wall Street Journal*, Sept. 16, 2003, D8.

44. Kate Zezima, "For Many, 'Washroom' Seems to Be Just a Name," *New York Times*, Sept. 13, 2010.

45. Ibid.

46. Ibid.

47. Ibid.

48. Maryellen E. Guinan, Maryanne McGuckin-Guinan, and Alice Sevareid,"Who Washes Hands after Using the Bathroom?" *American Journal of Infection Control* 25 (1997): 424–25.

49. Jyothi Thumma, Allison Aiello, and Betsy Foxman, "The Association between Handwashing Practices and Illness Symptoms among College Students Living in a University Dormitory," *American Journal of Infection Control* 37 (2009): 70–72.

50. Carl P. Borchgrevink, JaeMin Cha, and SeungHyun Kim, "Hand Washing Practices in a College Town Environment," *Journal of Environmental Health* 75 (2013): 18–24.

51. Ibid.

52. J. M. Schulte, L. Williams, J. Asghar, T. Dang, S. Bedwell, K. Guerrero, D. Hamaker, S. Stonecipher, J. Zoretic, and C. Chow, "How We Didn't Clean Up until We Washed Our Hands: Shigellosis in an Elementary and Middle School in North Texas," *Southern Medical Journal* 105 (2012): 1–4.

53. V. Curtis and S. Cairncross, "Effect of Washing Hands with Soap on Diarrhoea Risk in the Community: A Systematic Review," *Lancet Infectious Diseases* 3 (2003): 275–81.

54. Allison E. Aiello, Rebecca M. Coulborn, Vanessa Perez, and Elaine L. Larson, "Effect of Hand Hygiene on Infectious Disease Risk in the Community Setting: A Meta-Analysis," *American Journal of Public Health* 98 (2008): 1372–81.

55. Charlotte Warren-Gash, Ellen Fragaszy, and Andrew C. Hayward, "Hand Hygiene to Reduce Community Transmission of Influenza and Acute Respiratory Tract Infection: A Systematic Review," *Influenza and Other Respiratory Viruses* 7 (2012): 738–49.

56. Maxine Burton, Emma Cobb, Peter Donachie, Gaby Judah, Val Curtis, and Wolf-Peter Schmidt, "The Effect of Handwashing with Water or Soap on Bacterial

Contamination of Hands," *International Journal of Environmental Research and Public Health* 8 (2011): 97–104.

57. Stephen P. Luby, Amal K. Halder, Tarique Huda, Leanne Unicomb, and Richard B. Johnston, "The Effect of Handwashing at Recommended Times with Water Alone and with Soap on Child Diarrhea in Rural Bangladesh: An Observational Study," *PLOS Medicine* 8 (2011): 1–12.

58. R. N. Hiremath, A. Kotwal, R. Kunte, S. V. Hiremath, and Venkatesh, "Hand Washing with Soap: The Most Effective 'Do-It-Yourself' Vaccine?" *National Journal of Community Medicine* 3 (2012): 551–54.

59. Department of Health and Human Services, Food and Drug Administration, "Safety and Effectiveness of Consumer Antiseptics," *Federal Register* 78, no. 242 (Dec. 17, 2013): 76444–71. http://www.gpo.gov/fdsys/pkg/FR-2013-12-17/pdf/2013 -29814.pdf.

60. Matthew Perrone, "Decades-Old Question: Is Antibacterial Soap Safe?" *Seattle Times*, May 2, 2013.

61. Heather Buschman, "The Dirty Side of Soap," University of San Diego Health System Newsroom, Nov. 13, 2014. http://health.ucsd.edu/news/releases/pages/2014 -11-17-dirty-side-of-soap.aspx. See also *Federal Register*, 76444–71.

62. Ibid.

63. Siamak P. Yazdankhah, Anne A. Scheie, E. Arne Hoiby, Bjorn-Tore Lunestad, Even Heir, Tor Oystein Fotland, Kristine Naterstad, and Hilde Kruse, "Triclosan and Antimicrobial Resistance in Bacteria: An Overview," *Microbial Drug Resistance* 12 (2006): 83–90.

64. Coco Ballantyne, "Do Antibacterial Soaps Do More Harm Than Good?" *Scientific American*, February 2008, p. 96. http://www.scientificamerican.com/article /fact-or-fiction-2008-02/.

65. Mei-Fei Yueh, Koji Taniguchi, Shujuan Chen, Ronald M. Evans, Bruce D. Hammock, Michael Karin, and Robert Tukey, "The Commonly Used Antimicrobial Additive Triclosan Is a Liver Tumor Promoter," *Proceedings of the National Academy of Sciences* 111 (2014): 17200–05.

66. *Federal Register*, 76444–71.

67. Steve Karnowski, "Minnesota Becomes First State to Ban Antibacterial Chemical Triclosan from Soaps," *Huffington Post*, May 20, 2014. www.huffington-post.com/2014/05/20/minnesota-ban-triclosan-antibacterial-soap_n_5357733 .html.

68. Ballantyne, "Do Antibacterial Soaps Do More Harm Than Good?"

69. P. Anuradha, P. Yasoda Devi, and M. S. Prakash, "Effect of Handwashing Agents on Bacterial Contamination," *Indian Journal of Pediatrics* 66 (1999): 7–10.

70. B. A. Hoque and A. Briend, "A Comparison of Local Handwashing Agents in Bangladesh," *American Journal of Tropical Medicine and Hygiene* 94 (1991): 61–64.

71. Sally Bloomfield and Kumar Jyoti Nath, "Use of Ash and Mud for Hand-washing in Low Income Communities: International Scientific Forum on Home Hygiene (IFH) Expert Review," October 2009. http://www.ifh-homehygiene.org.

72. A. J. Pickering, A. B. Boehm, M. Mwanjali, and J. Davis, "Efficacy of Water-less Hand Hygiene Compared with Handwashing with Soap: A Field Study in Dar es Salaam, Tanzania," *American Journal of Tropical Medicine and Hygiene* 82 (2010): 270–78.

73. Ibid.

74. Ibid.

75. A. J. Pickering, J. Davis, and A. B. Boehm, "Efficacy of Alcohol-Based Hand Sanitizer on Hands Soiled with Dirt and Cooking Oil," *Journal of Water and Health* 9 (2011): 429–33.

76. M. T. Oughton, V. G. Loo, N. Dendukuri, S. Fenn, and M. D. Libman, "Hand Hygiene with Soap and Water Is Superior to Alcohol Rub and Antiseptic Wipes for Removal of *Clostridium difficile*," *Infection Control and Hospital Epidemiology* 30 (2009): 939–44.

77. Ibid.

78. U. Jabbar, J. Leischner, D. Kasper, R. Gerber, S. P. Sambol, J. P. Parada, S. Johnson, and D. N. Gerding, "Effectiveness of Alcohol-Based Hand Rubs for Re-moval of Clostridium Difficile Spores from Hands," *Infection Control and Hospital Epidemiology* 31 (2010): 565–70.

79. Bruce Hammond, Yusuf Ali, Eleanor Fendler, Michael Dolan, and Sandra Donovan, "Effect of Hand Sanitizer Use on Elementary School Absenteeism," *American Journal of Infection Control* 28 (2000) 340–46.

80. Cindy White, Robin Kolbie, Rebecca Carlson, Natasha Lipson, Mike Dolan, Yusuf Ali, and Mojee Cline, "The Effect of Hand Hygiene on Illness Rate Among Students in University Dorms," *American Journal of Infection Control* 31 (2003): 364–70.

81. Grace M. Lee, Joshua A. Salomon, Jennifer F. Friedman, Patricia L. Hibberd, Dennis Ross-Degnan, Eva Zasloff, Sitso Bediako, and Donald A. Goldmann, "Ill-ness Transmission in the Home: A Possible Role for Alcohol-Based Hand Gels," *Pediatrics* 115 (2005): 852–60.

82. Ibid.

83. *WHO Guidelines on Hand Hygiene in Healthcare: First Global Patient Safety Challenge/Clean Care Is Safer Care* (Geneva: World Health Organization, 2009).

84. Ibid., 152.

85. Ibid.

86. American Academy of Pediatrics, American Public Health Association, and National Resource Center for Health and Safety in Child Care and Early Education, *Caring for Our Children: National Health and Safety Performance Standards: Guide-*

lines for Early Care and Education Programs, 3rd ed. (Elk Grove Village, IL: American Academy of Pediatrics; Washington, DC: American Public Health Association, 2011). Also available at http://nrckids.org.

87. Ibid., Standard 3.2.2.2, "Handwashing Procedure," 111.

88. http://www.today.com/home/how-often-should-you-wash-bath-towels -1D80418474.

89. Keith Redway and Shameem Fawdar, "A Comparative Study of Three Different Hand Drying Methods: Paper Towel, Warm Air Dryer, Jet Air Dryer" (paper presented at the European Tissue Symposium, Brussels, November 2008). http://www.cleanlink.com/pdf/casestudieswhitepapers/ETS030609.pdf.

90. Percentage (%) dryness = (weight of water on undried hands – weight of water on dried hands) ÷ (weight of water on undried hands) × 100.

91. Redway and Fawdar, "A Comparative Study."

92. Ibid.

93. Ibid.

94. Ibid.

95. E. Margas, E. Maguire, C. R. Berland, F. Welander, and J. T. Holah, "Assessment of the Environmental Microbiological Cross Contamination Following Hand Drying with Paper Hand Towels or an Air Blade Dryer," *Journal of Applied Microbiology* 115 (2013): 572–82.

96. http://www.sca.com/en/About_SCA/SCAs-business-and-operations -worldwide/Tissue/.

97. Cunrui Huang, Wenjun Ma, and Susan Stack, "The Hygienic Efficacy of Different Hand-Drying Methods: A Review of the Evidence," *Mayo Clinic Proceedings* 87 (2012): 791–98.

98. Ibid.

99. Ibid.

100. Ibid.

2. Microbe Hunting: Historic and Biological Roots of Hygiene

1. Talmud *Berachot* 14b

2. Talmud *Eiruvin* 21b

3. Thomas H. Maugh II, "Dead Sea Scrolls Reveal a Tragic Irony," *Record*, November 16, 2006, A-20.

4. Matthew Henry, *Exposition of the Old and New Testaments*, 6 vols. (1708–1710). Sacred Texts Archive, http://www.sacred-texts.com/bib/cmt/henry/index.htm. Henry was a Welsh Presbyterian minister who lived from 1662–1714.

5. Talmud *Sotah* 4b. Note that the written Babylonian Talmud was completed about five centuries after the death of Jesus Christ, in the diaspora Jewish commu-

nity of Babylonia. It was a formalized record of rabbinic discussions based on oral tradition handed down from Moses.

6. John Gill, *Exposition on the New Testament*, 3 vols. (1746–1748). Sacred Texts Archive, http://www.sacred-texts.com/bib/cmt/gill/index.htm. John Gill was an English Baptist pastor, Biblical scholar, and theologian, who lived from 1697–1771 and mastered Greek and Hebrew, along with logic and other disciplines.

7. Greek Orthodox Archdiocese of America. http://www.goarch.org/chapel/liturgical_texts/baptism.

8. *WHO Guidelines on Hand Hygiene in Health Care* (Geneva: World Health Organization, 2009), 79.

9. Ibid.

10. Robert E. Adler, *Medical Firsts from Hippocrates to the Human Genome* (Hoboken, NJ: John Wiley, 2004), 36–40.

11. Mohammed ibn Hasan ibn Ali Abu Ja'far al-Tusi, *A Concise Description of Islamic Law and Legal Opinion*, trans. A. Ezzati (London: ICAS Press, 2008), 1–8.

12. Ibid., 3–4.

13. Ibid., 6.

14. Ibid., 8.

15. Ibid., 1–44.

16. Tamar Lewin, "Some U.S. Universities Install Foot Baths for Muslim Students," *New York Times*, August 7, 2007.

17. Bahá'u'lláh, *The Kitab-i-Aqdas: The Most Holy Book*. http://www.bahai.org/library/authoritative-texts/bahaullah/kitab-i-aqdas/#f=f10-582.

18. "Living Waters: The Daily Baha'i Obligatory Prayers: Ablutions." http://obligatoryprayers.blogspot.com/2009/01/ablutions.html#.vNktYsI5BMs.

19. Philip M. Tierno Jr. *The Secret Life of Germs* (New York: Pocket Books, 2001), 20.

20. J. Singh, M. S. Desai, C. S. Pandav, and S. P. Desai, "Contributions of Ancient Indian Physicians—Implications for Modern Times," *Journal of Postgraduate Medicine* 58 (2012): 73–78.

21. Ibid.

22. B. A. Hoque and A. Brand,"A Comparison of Local Handwashing Agents in Bangladesh," *Journal of Tropical Medicine and Hygiene* 94 (1991): 61–64.

23. *WHO Guidelines*, 2009, 83.

24. Ibid., 79.

25. Ibid.

26. http://www.religionresourcesonline.org/religious-beliefs-wiki/Summary_of_shintoism.

27. http://www.onmarkproductions.com/html/shinto-deities.html#suijin.

28. Allison E. Aiello, Rebecca M. Coulborn, Vanessa Perez, and Elaine L. Larson, "Effect of Hand Hygiene on Infectious Disease Risk in the Community Setting: A Meta-Analysis," *American Journal of Public Health* 98 (2008): 1372–81.

29. Stephen P. Luby, Amal K. Halder, Tarique Huda, Leanne Unicomb, and Richard B. Johnson, "The Effect of Handwashing at Recommended Times with Water Alone and with Soap on Child Diarrhea in Rural Bangladesh: An Observational Study," *PLOS Medicine* 8 (2011): e1001052, doi:10.1371/journal.pmed.1001052.

30. Ibid.

31. Maxine Burton, Emma Cobb, Peter Donachie, Gaby Judah, Val Curtis, and Wolf-Peter Schmidt, "The Effect of Handwashing with Water or Soap on Bacterial Contamination of Hands," *International Journal of Environmental Research and Public Health* 8 (2011): 97–104.

32. Virginia Smith, *Clean: A History of Personal Hygiene and Purity* (New York: Oxford University Press, 2007), 74–101.

33. Manolis J. Papagrigorakis, Christos Yapijakis, Philippos N. Synodinos, and Effie Baziotopoulou-Valavani, "DNA Examination of Ancient Dental Pulp Incriminates Typhoid Fever as a Probable Cause of the Plague of Athens," *International Journal of Infectious Diseases* 10 (2006): 206–14.

34. Dorothy H. Crawford, *Deadly Companions* (New York: Oxford University Press, 2007), 77.

35. Ibid., 77–79.

36. Smith, *Clean*, 106.

37. Crawford, *Deadly Companions*, 79–81.

38. Tierno, *The Secret Life of Germs*, 21.

39. Crawford, *Deadly Companions*, 85.

40. Ibid., 82.

41. Virginia Iommi Echeverria, "Girolamo Fracastoro and the Invention of Syphilis," *Historia, Ciencias, Saude-Manguinhos (Rio de Janeiro)* 17 (2010): 877–84.

42. Paul de Kruif, *Microbe Hunters* (New York: Pocket Books, 1964), 1. (The first edition of this classic was published by Harcourt Brace in 1926.)

43. Ibid., 8.

44. Abstract of "Letter from Mr. Anthony Leevvenhoeck at Delft, dated Sep. 17, 1683. Containing Microscopical Observations about Animals in the Scrurf of the Teeth," *Philosophical Transactions of the Royal Society of London* 14, no. 159 (May 20, 1684): 568–74, as quoted in Thomas D. Brock, *Milestones in Microbiology: 1546 to 1940* (Washington, DC: American Society of Microbiology, 1999), 9–10.

45. De Kruif, *Microbe Hunters*, 9–22.

46. Lazaro Spallanzani, *Tracts on the Nature of Animals and Vegetables* (Edinburgh: William Creech and Ar. Constable, 1799), as cited in Brock, *Milestones in Microbiology*, 13–15.

47. Ibid., 22–52.

48. Adler, *Medical Firsts*, 95–98.

49. Ibid., 95.

50. Ignaz Semmelweis, "Vortrag uber die Genesis des Puerperalfiebers" (Lecture on the genesis of puerperal fever), *Protokoll der allgemeinen Versammlund der k.k. Gesellschaft der Aerzte zu Wien*, May 15, 1850, as quoted in Brock, *Milestones in Microbiology*, 80–82.

51. Adler, *Medical Firsts*, 98.

52. Ibid., 98–100.

53. De Kruif, *Microbe Hunters*, 53–65.

54. Charles Cagniard-Latour, "Memoire sur la fermentation vineuse," *Annales de chimie et de physique* 68 (1838), 206–22, as quoted in Brock, *Milestones in Microbiology*, 23.

55. De Kruif, *Microbe Hunters*, 53–65.

56. Ibid.

57. Louis Pasteur, "Memoire sur les corpuscles organizes qui existent dans l'atmosphere. Examen de la doctrine des generations spontanees," *Annales des sciences naturelles*, 4th ser., vol. 16 (1861), 5–98, as quoted in Brock, *Milestones in Microbiology*, 43–48.

58. Joseph Lister, "On the Antiseptic Principle in the Practice of Surgery," *British Medical Journal* 2 (1867): 246–48.

59. https://www.listerine.com/mouthwash/antiseptic/listerine-original-mouthwash.

60. De Kruif, *Microbe Hunters*, 95.

61. Tierno, *Secret Life of Germs*, 62–63.

62. Brock, *Milestones in Microbiology*, 89–118.

63. Adler, *Medical Firsts*, 76–82.

64. Brock, *Milestones in Microbiology*, 23.

65. Centers for Disease Control and Prevention, "Estimates of Deaths Associated with Seasonal Influenza—United States, 1976–2007," *Morbidity and Mortality Weekly Report* 59 (2010): 1057–62.

3. First Do No Harm

1. http://www.WHO.int/gho and mchb.hrsa.gov/chusa13/perinatal-health-statistics.

2. http://www.cancer.gov/dictionary?cdrid=346525 and www.medicinenet.com/script/main/art.asp?articlekey=33263.

3. Ralph Peeples, Catherine T. Harris, and Thomas B. Metzloff, "The Process of Managing Medical Malpractice Cases: The Role of Standard of Care," *Wake Forest Law Review* 37 (2002): 877.

4. "Trials of War Criminals before the Nuremberg Military Tribunals under Control Council Law No. 10," in *Nuremberg Code*, vol. 2 (Washington, DC: U.S. Government Printing Office, 1949), 181–82. Archived at U.S. Department of Health and Human Services, Office for Human Research Protections. http://www.hhs.gov /ohrp/archive/nurcode.html.

5. Tom L. Beauchamp and James F. Childress, *Principles of Biomedical Ethics*, 7th ed. (New York: Oxford University Press, 2012).

6. John T. James, "A New, Evidence–Based Estimate of Patient Harms Associated with Hospital Care," *Journal of Patient Safety* 9 (2013): 122–28.

7. Centers for Disease Control and Prevention, Healthcare-Associated Infection (HAI) Prevalence Survey data, 2011. www.cdc.gov/HAI/surveillance.

8. Dror Cantrell, Oded Shamriz, Matan J. Cohen, Zvi Stern, Colin Block, and Mayer Brezis, "Hand Hygiene Compliance by Physicians: Marked Heterogeneity due to Local Culture?" *American Journal of Infection Control* 37 (2009): 301–5.

9. http://www.WHO.int/gho and mchb.hrsa.gov/chusa13/perinatal-health -statistics.

10. The Vicks Formula 44 commercial in 1984 featured actor Chris Robinson, aka Dr. Rick Webber from *General Hospital*. He was replaced in the ad in 1986 by actor Peter Bergman, aka Dr. Cliff Warner of *All My Children*. You can view the latter advertisement on YouTube. Clearly, daytime soap opera doctors gain enough experience to practice virtual medicine on unsuspecting viewers, aka patients.

11. Cedars-Sinai Medical Center Guidelines: Infection Control Practices: Surgical Hand Scrub Procedure, Los Angeles, California, June 2008. https://www.cedars -sinai.edu/Patients/Programs-and-Services/Surgery/Documents/I12-Surg-Hand -Scrub-_2_-121945.pdf.

12. Ibid.

13. Miranda Suchomel, Walter Koller, Michael Kundi, and Manfred Rotter, "Surgical Hand Rub: Influence of Duration of Application on the Immediate and 3-Hours Effects of N-Propanol and Isopropanol," *American Journal of Infection Control* 37 (2009): 289–93.

14. Jean Jacques Parienti, Pascal Thibon, Remy Heller, Yannick LeRoux, Peter von Theobold, Herve Bensadoun, Alain Bouvet, Francois Lemarchand, and Xavier Le Coutour, "Hand-Rubbing with an Aqueous Alcoholic Solution vs. Traditional Surgical Hand-Scrubbing and 30-Day Surgical Site Infection Rates," *Journal of the American Medical Association* 288 (2002): 722–27.

15. Michael J. Messina, Lindsey A. Brodell, Robert T. Brodell, and Eliot N. Mostow, "Hand Hygiene in the Dermatologist's Office: To Wash or to Rub?" *Journal of the American Academy of Dermatology* 59 (2008): 1043–49.

16. Ibid.

17. Ibid.

18. K. Vagholkar and K. Julka, "Preoperative Skin Preparation: Which Is the Best Method?" *Internet Journal of Surgery* 28, no. 4 (2012). http://ispub.com/IJs /28/4/14353.

19. Maria Grazia Capretti, Fabrizio Sandri, Elisabetta Tridapalli, Silvia Galletti, Elisabetta Petracci, and Giacomo Faldella, "Impact of a Standardized Hand Hygiene Program on the Incidence of Nosocomial Infection in Very Low Birth Weight Infants," *American Journal of Infection Control* 36 (2008): 430–35.

20. Rezhan Hussein, Rashida Khakoo, and Gerald Hobbs, "Hand Hygiene Practices in Adult versus Pediatric Intensive Care Units at a University Hospital before and after Intervention," *Scandanavian Journal of Infectious Diseases* 39 (2007): 566–70.

21. Ibid.

22. Joan M. Duggan, Sandra Hensley, Sadik Khuder, Thomas J. Papadimos, and Lloyd Jacobs, "Inverse Correlation between Level of Professional Education and Rate of Handwashing Compliance in a Teaching Hospital," *Infection Control and Hospital Epidemiology* 29 (2008): 534–38.

23. Messina et al., "Hand Hygiene in the Dermatologist's Office."

24. Chris Gonzalez, Timothy Averch, Lee Ann Boyd, J. Quentin Clemens, Robert Dowling, Howard B. Goldman, Danil V. Makarov, Vic Senese, and Mary Anne Wasner, "AUA/SUNA White Paper on the Incidence, Prevention and Treatment of Complications Related to Prostate Needle Biopsy," American Urological Association, Linthicum, Maryland, 2012. https://www.auanet.org/common/pdf/practices -resources/quality/patient_safety/AUA-SUNA-PNBWhitePaper.pdf.

25. Ana M. Novoa, Teresa Pi-Sunyer, Maria Sala, Eduard Molins, and Xavier Castells, "Evaluation of Hand Hygiene Adherence in a Tertiary Hospital," *American Journal of Infection Control* 35 (2007): 676–83.

26. Ibid.

27. Mona M. Basurrah and Tariq A. Madani, "Handwashing and Gloving Practice among Health Care Workers in Medical and Surgical Wards in a Tertiary Care Centre in Riyadh, Saudi Arabia," *Scandinavian Journal of Infectious Diseases* 38 (2007): 620–24.

28. Luis Fernando Perez-Gonzalez, Juana Maria Ruiz-Gonzalez, and Daniel E. Noyola, "Nosocomial Bacteremia in Children: A 15-Year Experience at a General Hospital in Mexico," *Infection Control and Hospital Epidemiology* 28 (2007): 418–22.

29. Cantrell et al., "Hand Hygiene Compliance by Physicians."

30. Ibid.

31. Ibid.

32. Ibid.

33. Duggan et al., "Inverse Correlation Between Level of Professional Education."

34. Ibid.

35. Ibid.

36. Ruth M. Sladek, Malcolm J. Bond, and Paddy Phillips, "Why Don't Doctors Wash Their Hands? A Correlational Study of Thinking Styles and Hand Hygiene," *American Journal of Infection Control* 36 (2008): 399–406.

37. Ibid.

38. *Weight Watchers 360° Booklet* (2012); www.weightwatchers.com.

39. Cantrell et al., "Hand Hygiene Compliance by Physicians."

40. Michael Whitby, Mary-Louise McLaws, and Michael W. Ross, "Why Healthcare Workers Don't Wash Their Hands: A Behavioral Explanation," *Infection Control and Hospital Epidemiology* 27 (2006): 484–92.

41. E. A. Jenner, B. Fletcher, P. Watson, F. A. Jones, L. Miller, and G. M. Scott, "Discrepancy between Self-Reported and Observed Hand Hygiene Behaviour in Healthcare Professionals," *Journal of Hospital Infection* 63 (2006): 418–22.

42. Ibid.

43. Ibid.

44. Ibid.

45. Ibid.

46. Ibid.

47. Ibid.

48. Ibid.

49. Barbara I. Braun, Linda Kusek, and Elaine Larson, "Measuring Adherence to Hand Hygiene Guidelines: A Field Survey for Examples of Effective Practices," *American Journal of Infection Control* 37 (2009): 282–88.

50. Ibid.

51. Roni Caryn Rabin, "When the Surgeon Is Infected, How Safe Is the Surgery?" *New York Times*, July 3, 2007, F5.

52. Ibid.

53. Thomas J. Papadimos, "Unwashed Doctors," *International Journal of Critical Illness and Injury Science* 1 (2011): 87–88.

54. Ibid.

55. Guy J. Maddern, "The Surgical Scrub—Who Cares?" *ANZ Journal of Surgery* 74 (2004): 720.

56. Suzanne C. Gordon, "Ask Me If I Cleaned My Hands?" *Journal of the American Medical Association* 307 (2012): 1591–92.

57. Ibid.

58. Ibid.

4. Touch at Your Own Risk

1. Girolamo Fracastoro, *De Contagione, Contagiosis Morbis et eorum Ciratione* (*Contagion, Contagious Diseases and Their Treatment*), trans. Wilmer C. Wright

(1546; reprint, New York: G. P. Putnam's Sons, 1930); reprinted in: Thomas D. Brock, *Milestones in Microbiology: 1546–1940* (Washington, DC: ASM Press, 1999), 70.

2. Ibid., 71–72.

3. "My Cabbage," *Scrubs*, Season 5, Episode 12, February 28, 2006. http://www .imdb.com/title/tt0771285/.

4. Louis D. Brandeis, "What Publicity Can Do." *Harper's Weekly* 20 (1913).

5. Julie Deardorff, "The Five-Second Rule? Location, Not Time, Is Key," *Record*, August 2, 2010, F2.

6. Colin Steinlechner, Graeme Wilding, and N. Cumberland, "Microbes on Ties: Do They Correlate with Wound Infection?" *Annals of the Royal College of Surgeons of England*, supp. 84 (2002): 307–9.

7. Michael Day, "Doctors Are Told to Ditch 'Disease Spreading' Neckties," *British Medical Journal* 332 (2006): 442.

8. Pedro-Jose Lopez, Ori Ron, Prabha Parthasarathy, James Soothill, and Lewis Spitz, "Bacterial Counts from Hospital Doctors' Ties Are Higher Than Those from Shirts," *American Journal of Infection Control* 37 (2009): 79–80.

9. Miryam Wahrman, Brian Nelson, and Brianna McSweeney, "Can Neckties Make You Sick? Microbial Growth on Silk vs. Polyester" (paper presented at Research and Scholarship Day, William Paterson University, Wayne, New Jersey, April 7, 2011).

10. Ibid.

11. Miryam Z. Wahrman, Karina Kuruvilla, Shamil Javed, and Peter Rogers, "Microbial Contamination and Decontamination of Textiles" (paper presented at Research and Scholarship Day, William Paterson University, Wayne, New Jersey, April 5, 2012).

12. Ibid.

13. Ibid.

14. Ibid.

15. Alice N. Neely and Matthew P. Maley, "Survival of Enterococci and Staphylococci on Hospital Fabrics and Plastic," *Journal of Clinical Microbiology* 38 (2000): 724–26.

16. Miryam Z. Wahrman, Khushnuma Sabavala, Henry Raab, and Shalaka Paranjpe, "Growth, Adherence and Transfer of Bacteria on Textiles" (paper presented at Research and Scholarship Day, William Paterson University, Wayne, New Jersey, April 4, 2013).

17. *Health and Safety in the Child Care Setting: Prevention of Infectious Disease: A Curriculum for the Training of Child Care Providers*, mod. 1, 2nd ed. (Oakland, CA: California Child Care Health Program, 2001), 35–37. http://www.ucsfchildcare health.org/pdfs/Curricula/idc2book.pdf.

18. Daniel Smith, John Alverdy, Gary An, Maureen Coleman, Sylvia Garcia-Houchins, Jessica Green, Kevin Keegan, Scott T. Kelley, Benjamin C. Kirkup, Larry Kociolek, Hal Levin, Emily Landon, Paula Olsiewski, Rob Knight, Jeffrey Siegel, Stephen Weber, and Jack Gilbert, "The Hospital Microbiome Project: Meeting Report for the 1st Hospital Microbiome Project Workshop on Sampling Design and Building Science Measurements, Chicago, USA, June 7th–8th 2012," *Standards in Genomic Sciences* 8 (2013): 112–17.

19. *Health and Safety in the Child Care Setting*, 35–37.

20. Fredd Elliott, "Effective Encouragement," *Occupational Health and Safety* 77 (2008): 118–22.

21. Centers for Disease Control and Prevention estimate, 2014. http://www.cdc .gov/foodborneburden/.

22. Corey H. Basch, Laura A. Guerra, Zerlina MacDonald, Myladys Marte, and Charles E. Basch, "Glove Changing Habits in Mobile Food Vendors in New York City," *Journal of Community Health* 40, no. 4 (August 2015): 699–701, doi:10.1007 /s10900-014-9987-7.

23. Corey H. Basch, Miryam Z. Wahrman, Jay Shah, Laura A. Guerra, Zerlina MacDonald, Myladys Marte, and Charles E Basch, "Glove Changing When Handling Money: Observational and Microbiological Analysis," *Journal of Community Health*, published online October 13, 2015, doi:10.1007/s10900-015-0101-6.

24. Miryam Z. Wahrman and Henry Raab, "Survival and Transfer of Bacteria on Latex Gloves and Paper Currency," forthcoming.

25. H. K. Naver and F. Gottrup, "Incidence of Glove Perforations in Gastrointestinal Surgery and the Protective Effect of Double Gloves: A Prospective, Randomized Controlled Study," *European Journal of Surgery* 166 (2000): 293–95.

26. Gunter Kampf and Axel Kramer, "Epidemiologic Background of Hand Hygiene and Evaluation of the Most Important Agents for Scrubs and Rubs," *Clinical Microbiol Reviews* 17 (2004): 863–93.

27. Michael Barza, "Efficacy and Tolerability of ClO2-Generating Gloves," *Clinical Infectious Diseases* 38 (2004): 857–863.

28. "Treated Glove," *Occupational Health and Safety*, 74 (2005): 79.

29. Barry Michaels, "Handling Money and Serving Ready-to-Eat Food," *Food Service Technology* 2 (2002): 1–3.

30. Corey H. Basch et al., "Glove Changing When Handling Money."

31. Theodore W. Pope, Peter T. Ender, William K. Woelk, Michael A. Korosch, and Thomas M. Koroscil, "Bacterial Contamination of Paper Currency," *Southern Medical Journal* 95 (2002): 1408–10.

32. Debajit Borah, Prapap Parida, and Tarun Kumar, "Paper Currencies: A Potential Carrier of Pathogenic Microorganisms," *International Journal of Applied Biology and Pharmaceutical Technology* 3 (2012): 23–25.

33. Habip Gedik, Timothy Voss, and Andreas Voss, "Money and Transmission of Bacteria," *Antimicrobial Resistance and Infection Control* 2 (2013): 22, doi10.1186 /2047-2994-2-22.

34. A. P. Jepson, C. McDougall, A. Clark, A. Bateman, G. Williamson, and M. E. Kaufmann, "Finger Rings Should Be Removed Prior to Scrubbing," *Journal of Hospital Infection* 64 (2006): 197–98.

35. Inci Yildirim, Mehmet Ceyhan, Ali Bulent Cengiz, Arzu Bagdat, Cagri Barin, Tezer Kurluk, and Deniz Gur, "A Prospective Comparative Study of the Relationship Between Different Types of Rings and Microbial Hand Colonization among Pediatric Intensive Care Unit Nurses," *International Journal of Nursing Studies* 45 (2008): 1572–76.

36. G. Velvizhi, G. Anupriya, G. Sucilathangam, M. A. Ashihabegum, T. Jeyamuruga, and N. Palaniappan, "Wristwatches as the Potential Sources of Hospital-Acquired Infections," *Journal of Clinical and Diagnostic Research* 6 (2012): 807–10.

37. David Cressey, "Time for Doctors to Unstrap Their Watches?" *Nature* 3 (January 2008), doi:10.1038/news.2007.403.

38. Anne Gardner, "Deadly Pathogens Found on Lanyards," *Australian Nursing Journal* 15 (2008): 12.

39. Yves Longtin, Alexis Schneider, Clement Tschopp, Gesuele Renzi, Angele Gayet-Ageron, Jacques Schrenzel, and Didier Pittet, "Contamination of Stethoscopes and Physicians' Hands after a Physical Examination," *Mayo Clinic Proceedings* 89 (2014): 291–99. http://dx.doi.org/10.1016/j.mayocp.2013.11.016.

40. Dennis G. Maki, "Stethoscopes and Heath Care-Associated Infection," *Mayo Clinic Proceedings* 89 (2014): 277–79.

41. Margery Williams, *The Velveteen Rabbit, or How Toys Become Real*, illus. William Nicholson (New York: Doubleday, 1922).

42. Michael W. Milam, Melanie Hall, Teri Pringle, and Kay Buchanan, "Bacterial Contamination of Fabric Stethoscope Covers: The Velveteen Rabbit of Health Care?" *Infection Control and Hospital Epidemiology*, 22 (2001): 653–55.

43. R. R. W. Brady, J. Verran, N. N. Damani, and A. P. Gibb, "Review of Mobile Communication Devices as Potential Reservoirs of Nosocomial Pathogens," *Journal of Hospital Infection* 71 (2009): 295–300.

44. Ibid.

45. Yeon Joo Lee, Chul-Gyu Yoo, Choon-Taek Lee, Hee Soon Chung, Young Whan Kim, Sung Koo Han, and Jae-Joon Yim, "Contamination Rates Between Smart Cell Phones and Non-Smart Cell Phones of Healthcare Workers," *Journal of Hospital Medicine* 8 (2013): 144–47.

46. Lee M. Kiedrowski, Abhilash Perisetti, Mark H. Loock, Margaret L. Khaitsa, and Dubert M. Guerrero, "Disinfection of iPad to Reduce Contamination with *Clostridium difficile* and Methicillin-Resistant *Staphylococcus aureus*," *American Journal of Infection Control* 41 (2013): 1136–37.

47. Kate Murphy, "Cleaning the Mobile Germ Warehouse," *New York Times*, Jan. 1, 2014.

48. Gardiner Harris, "When the Mango Bites Back," *New York Times*, August 27, 2012.

49. Andrew E. Waters, Tania Contente-Cuomo, Jordan Buchhagen, Cindy M. Liu, Lindsey Watson, Kimberly Pearce, Jeffrey T. Forster, Jolene Bowers, Elizabeth M. Driebe, David M. Engelthaler, Paul S. Keim, and Lance B. Price, "Multidrug-Resistant *Staphylococcus aureus* in U.S. Meat and Poultry," *Clinical Infectious Diseases* 52 (2011): 1227–30.

50. Annette Pruss-Ustun, Jamie Bartram, Thomas Clasen, John M. Colford, Jr., Oliver Cumming, Valerie Curtis, Sophie Bonjour, Alan D. Dangour, Jennifer De France, Lorna Fewtrell, Matthew C. Freeman, Bruce Gordon, Paul R. Hunter, Richard B. Johnston, Colin Mathers, Daniel Mausezahl, Kate Medlicott, Maria Neira, Meredith Stocks, Jennyfer Wolf, and Sandy Cairncross, "Burden of Disease from Inadequate Water, Sanitation and Hygiene in Low- and Middle-Income Settings: A Retrospective Analysis of Data from 145 Countries," *Tropical Medicine and International Health* 19 (2014): 894–905.

51. Matthew C. Freeman, Meredith E. Stocks, Oliver Cumming, Aurelie Jeandron, Julian P. T. Higgins, Jennyfer Wolf, Annette Pruss-Ustun, Sophie Bonjour, Paul R. Hunter, Lorna Fewtrell, and Valerie Curtis, "Hygiene and Health: Systematic Review of Handwashing Practices Worldwide and Update of Health Effects," *Tropical Medicine and International Health* 19 (2014): 906–16.

52. Centers for Disease Control and Prevention, "Travelers' Health: Destinations." http://wwwnc.cdc.gov/travel/destinations/list.

53. Morris Fishbein, *The Medical Follies* (New York: Boni and Liveright, 1925), 128–29.

54. "Sheets in Texas Beds Must Be 9 Feet Long," *San Francisco Call*, July 15, 1907, 9.

55. Mary Phillips, "The 9-Foot Bed Sheet," *Archivist*, August 29, 2009. http://newsok.com/the-9-foot-bed-sheet/article/3849647.

56. Fishbein, *Medical Follies*, 129.

57. Jill Schensul, "Traveling Healthy," *Record*, December 15, 2013, T-1.

58. Ibid.

59. Ibid.

60. Ibid.

61. Ibid.

5. Solutions: Protecting Ourselves and Society

1. Matthew C. Freeman, Meredith E. Stocks, Oliver Cumming, Aurelie Jeandron, Julian P. T. Higgins, Jennyfer Wolf, Annette Pruss-Ustun, Sophie Bonjour, Paul R. Hunter, Lorna Fewtrell, and Valerie Curtis, "Hygiene and Health: Systematic Re-

view of Handwashing Practices Worldwide and Update of Health Effects," *Tropical Medicine and International Health* 19 (2014): 906–16.

2. Ibid.

3. Jyothi Thumma, Allison Aiello, and Betsy Foxman, "The Association between Handwashing Practices and Illness Symptoms among College Students Living in a University Dormitory," *American Journal of Infection Control* 37 (2009): 70–72.

4. Kelly R. Reveles, Grace C. Lee, Natalie K. Boyd, and Cristopher R. Frei, "The Rise in *Clostridium difficile* Infection Incidence among Hospitalized Adults in the United States: 2001–2010," *American Journal of Infection Control* 42 (2014): 1028–32.

5. J. J. Parienti, P. Thibon, R. Heller, Y. LeRoux, P. von Theobold, H. Bensadoun, A. Bouvet, F. Lemarchand, and X. Le Coutour, "Hand-Rubbing with an Aqueous Alcoholic Solution vs Traditional Surgical Hand-Scrubbing and 30-Day Surgical Site Infection Rates," *Journal of the American Medical Association* 288 (2002): 722–27.

6. Sarah L. Edmunds, James Mann, Robert R. McCormack, David R. Macinga, Christopher M. Fricker, James W. Arbogast, and Michael J. Dolan, "SaniTwice: A Novel Approach to Hand Hygiene for Reducing Bacterial Contamination on Hands When Soap and Water Are Unavailable," *Journal of Food Protection* 73 (2010): 2296–2300.

7. Mark Sklansky, Nikhil Nadkami, and Lynn Ramirez-Avila, "Banning the Handshake from the Health Care Setting," *Journal of the American Medical Association* 311 (2014): 2477–78.

8. Leila I. Given, "The Bacterial Significance of the Handshake," *American Journal of Nursing* 29 (1929): 254–56.

9. Morton Hamburger Jr., "Transfer of Beta Hemolytic Streptococci by Shaking Hands," *American Journal of Medicine* 2 (1947): 23–25.

10. David Bishai, Liang Liu, Stephanie Shiau, Harrison Wang, Cindy Tsai, Margaret Liao, Shivaani Prakash, and Tracy Howard, "Quantifying School Officials' Exposure to Bacterial Pathogens at Graduation Ceremonies Using Repeated Observational Measures," *Journal of School Nursing* 27 (2011): 219–24.

11. Tamer Rabie and Valerie Curtis, "Handwashing and Risk of Respiratory Infections: A Quantitative Systematic Review," *Tropical Medicine and International Health* 11 (2006): 258–67.

12. Sara Mela and David Whitworth, "The Fist Bump: A More Hygienic Alternative to the Handshake," *American Journal of Infection Control* 42 (2014): 916–17.

13. Denise Liberty, personal communication.

14. Sklansky, "Banning the Handshake from the Health Care Setting."

15. Ibid.

16. Ibid.

17. Centers for Disease Control and Prevention, "Handwashing: Clean Hands Save Lives." http://www.cdc.gov/handwashing/.

18. World Health Organization, "Clean Hands Protect Against Infection." http://www.who.int/gpsc/clean_hands_protection/en/.

19. http://www.who.int/gpsc/tools/Five_moments/en/.

20. Ibid.

21. http://www.who.int/gpsc/en.

22. Joint Commission, *Measuring Hand Hygiene Adherence: Overcoming the Challenges* (Oakbrook Terrace, IL: Joint Commission, 2009).

23. Ibid., xv.

24. Ibid., xviii–xix.

25. Laszlo Szilagyi, Tamas Haidegger, Akos Lehotsky, Melinda Nagy, Erik-Artur Csonka, Xiuying Sun, Kooi Li Ooi, and Dale Fisher, "A Large-Scale Assessment of Hand Hygiene Quality and the Effectiveness of the 'WHO 6-Steps,'" *BMC Infectious Diseases* 13 (2013): 1–10.

26. "Promoting Hand Hygiene," *American Nurse* 40 (2008): 15.

27. Marin Schweizer, Heather Schacht Reisinger, Michael Ohl, Michelle B. Formanek, Amy Blevins, Melissa Ward, and Eli Perencevich, "Searching for an Optimal Hand Hygiene Bundle: A Meta-analysis," *Clinical Infectious Diseases* 58 (2014): 248–59.

28. Lucy Yardley, Sascha Miller, Wolff Schlotz, and Paul Little, "Evaluation of a Web-Based Intervention to Promote Hand Hygiene: Exploratory Randomized Controlled Trial," *Journal of Medical Internet Research* 13 (2011): e107, doi:10.2196/jmir.1963.

29. Bio-RiteAR. www.bio-rite.com.

30. HandyMD, Surewash; Interactive Entertainment Technology, Trinity College, Dublin.

31. Michelle Snow, George L. White Jr., and Han S. Kim, "Inexpensive and Time-Efficient Hand Hygiene Interventions Increase Elementary School Children's Hand Hygiene Rates," *Journal of School Health* 78 (2008): 230–33.

32. Richard Rogers and Oscar Hammerstein II, "You've Got to Be Carefully Taught," *South Pacific* (musical), 1949.

33. http://www.HenrytheHand.com.

34. Ibid.

35. James Gorman, "Survival's Ick Factor," *New York Times*, January 24, 2012, S1.

36. James F. Thrasher, Matthew J. Carpenter, Jeannette O. Andrews, Kevin M. Gray, Anthony J. Alberg, Ashley Navarro, Daniela B. Friedman, and Michael Cummings, "Cigarette Warning Label Policy Alternatives and Smoking-Related Health Disparities," *American Journal of Preventive Medicine* 43 (2012): 590–600.

37. Valerie A. Curtis, "A Natural History of Hygiene," *Canadian Journal of Infectious Disease and Medical Microbiology* 18 (2007): 11–14.

38. Valerie Curtis, "Why Disgust Matters," *Philosophical Transactions of the Royal Society B* 366 (2011): 3478–90.

39. Megan Oaten, Richard Stevenson, Paul Wagland, Trevor Case, and Betty Repacholi, "Parent-Child Transmission of Disgust and Hand Hygiene: The Role of Vocalizations, Gestures and Other Parental Responses," *Psychological Record* 64 (2014): 803–11.

40. Gaby Judah, Robert Aunger, Wolf-Peter Schmidt, Susan Michie, Stewart Granger, and Val Curtis, "Experimental Pretesting of Hand-Washing Interventions in a Natural Setting," *American Journal of Public Health* 99 (2009): S405–S411.

41. Janet E. Squires, Kathryn N. Suh, Stefanie Linklater, Natalie Bruce, Kathleen Gartke, Ian D. Graham, Alan Karovitch, Joanne Read, Virginia Roth, Karen Stockton, Emma Tibbo, Kent Woodhall, Jim Worthington, and Jeremy M. Grimshaw, "Improving Physician Hand Hygiene Compliance Using Behavioural Theories: A Study Protocol," *Implementation Science* 8 (2013): 16, doi:10.1186/1748-5908-8-16.

42. Ibid.

43. Janet E. Squires, Stefanie Linklater, Jeremy M. Grinshaw, Ian D. Graham, Katrina Sullivan, Natalie Bruce, Kathleen Gartke, Alan Karovitch, Virginia Roth, Karen Stockton, John Trickett, Jim Worthington, and Kathryn N. Suh, "Understanding Practice: Factors That Influence Physician Hand Hygiene Compliance," *Infection Control and Hospital Epidemiology* 35 (2014): 1511–20.

44. Ibid.

45. Occam's razor, also known as Ockham's razor, is a principle developed by the fourteenth-century Franciscan friar and philosopher William of Ockham (England), who reasoned that one should opt for the simplest explanation, with the fewest possible variables or causes.

46. Matthijs Boog, Vicki Erasmus, Jitske de Graaf, Elise van Beeck, Marijke Melles, and Ed van Beeck, "Assessing the Optimal Location for Alcohol-Based Hand Rub Dispensers in a Patient Room in an Intensive Care Unit," *BMC Infectious Diseases* 13 (2013): 1–17.

47. Marian Pokrywka, Jody Feigel, Barbara Douglas, Susan Crossberger, Amelia Hensler, and David Weber, "A Bundle Strategy Including Patient Hand Hygiene to Decrease *Clostridium difficile* Infections," *MedSurg Nursing* 23 (2014): 145–64.

48. Eleanor Smith, "Better Hygiene through Humiliation," *Atlantic* 314 (2014): 22.

49. http://www.biovigilsystems.com.

50. Ibid.

51. Ibid.

52. T. R. Lied and V. A. Kazandjian, "A Hawthorne Strategy: Implications for Performance Measurement and Improvement," *Clinical Performance and Quality Health Care* 6 (1998): 201–204.

53. Vincent C. C. Cheng, Josepha W. M. Tai, Sara K. Y. Ho, Jasper F. W. Chan, Kwan Ngai Hung, Pak Leung Ho, and Kwok Yung Yuen, "Introduction of an Electronic Monitoring System for Monitoring Compliance with Moments 1 and 4 of the WHO 'My 5 Moments for Hand Hygiene' Methodology," *BMC Infectious Diseases* 11 (2011): 151. http://www.biomedcentral.com/1471-2334/11/151.

54. Ibid.

55. Carolyn H. Dawson, and Jamie B. Mackrill, "Review of Technologies Available to Improve Hand Hygiene Compliance—Are They Fit for Purpose?" *Journal of Infection Prevention* 15 (2014): 222–28.

56. Tasmin Snow, "Weighing of Soap Dispenser Bags Sees Staff Handwashing Rates Soar," *Nursing Standard* 22 (2008): 11.

57. Jane Brown, Sue Szczepanska, Esther Tantan, and Julie Clark, "A Step Too far?" *Nursing Standard* 22 (2008): 4.

58. Simone Scheithauer, Vanessa Kamerseder, Peter Petersen, Jorg Christian Brokmann, Luis-Alberto Lopez-Gonzalez, Carsten Mach, Roland Schulze-Robbecke, and Sebastian W. Lemmen, "Improving Hand Hygiene Compliance in the Emergency Department: Getting to the Point," *BMC Infectious Diseases* 13 (2013): 367, doi:10.1186/1471-2334-13-367.

59. Centers for Disease Control and Prevention, "Handwashing: Clean Hands Save Lives." http://www.cdc.gov/handwashing/.

60. Morris Fishbein, *The Medical Follies* (New York: Boni and Liveright, 1925), 128–29.

61. 101 STAT. 1330 PUBLIC LAW 100-203—December 22, 1987.

62. US Food and Drug Administration, Food Code 2013, report no. PB2013-110462 (Alexandria, VA: US Department of Commerce, 2013). http://www.fda .gov/downloads/Food/GuidanceRegulation/RetailFoodProtection/FoodCode /UCM374510.pdf.

63. Ibid.

64. Ibid., sect. 2-201.12, 35.

65. Ibid., sect. 2–3, 46–50.

66. New York City Board of Health, *Health Code and Rules, 2015.* http://www.nyc .gov/html/doh/html/about/health-code.shtml.

67. Brady Dennis, "Widening Superbug Outbreak Raises Questions for FDA, Manufacturers," *Washington Post*, March 5, 2015.

68. Center for Devices and Radiological Health, Food and Drug Administration, "Reprocessing Medical Devices in Health Care Settings: Validation Methods and Labeling: Guidance for Industry and Food and Drug Administration Staff" (Rockville, MD: U.S. Department of Health and Human Services, March 17, 2015). http://www.fda.gov/downloads/MedicalDevices/DeviceRegulationandGuidance /GuidanceDocuments/UCM253010.pdf.

69. J. I. Allen, M. O. Allen, M. M. Olson, D. N. Gerding, C. J. Shanholzer, P. B. Meier, J. A. Vennes, and S. E. Silvis, "Pseudomonas Infection of the Biliary System Resulting from Use of a Contaminated Endoscope," *Gastroenterology* 92 (1987): 759–63.

70. Center for Devices and Radiological Health, "Reprocessing Medical Devices."

6. The Future of Hand Hygiene: It's Not a Game

1. Team Z-Man Games, "Pandemic," designer Matt Leacock (Rigaud, Quebec: Z-Man Games, 2012). www.zmangames.com.

2. Bill Hesselmar, Fei Sjoberg, Robert Saalman, Nils Aberg, Ingegerd Adlerberth, and Agnes E. Wold, "Pacifier Cleaning Practices and Risk of Allergy Development," *Pediatrics* 131 (2013): 1–9, doi: 10.1542/peds.2012-3345.

3. Mary van Kesteren, Basil G. Bibby, and George Packer Berry, "Studies on the Antibacterial Factors of Human Saliva," *Journal of Bacteriology* 43 (1942): 573–83.

4. B. L. Hart and K. L. Powell, "Antibacterial Properties of Saliva: Role in Maternal Periparturient Grooming and in Licking Wounds," *Physiology of Behavior* 48 (1990): 383–86.

5. Menno J. Oudhoff, Jan G. M. Bolscher, Kamran Nazmi, Hakan Kalay, Wim van't Hof, Arie V. Niew Amerongen, and Enno C. I. Veerman, "Histatins Are the Major Wound-Closure Stimulating Factors in Human Saliva as Identified in a Cell Culture Assay," *FASEB Journal* 22 (2008): 3805–12.

6. Michael Pollan, "Some of My Best Friends Are Bacteria," *New York Times Magazine*, May 19, 2013, 36.

7. Ibid.

8. Rachel Nolan, "Behind the Cover Story: Michael Pollan on Why Bacteria Aren't the Enemy," May 20, 2013. http://6thfloor.blogs.nytimes.com/2013/05/20 /behind-the-cover-story-michael-pollan-on-why-b.

9. Peter Andrey Smith, "A New Kind of Transplant Bank," *New York Times*, February 17, 2014.

10. Gina Kolata, "The New Generation of Microbe Hunters," *New York Times*, August 29, 2011.

11. Executive Office of the President, President's Council of Advisors on Science and Technology, *Report to the President on Combating Antibiotic Resistance* (Washington, DC: PCAST, September 2014). https://www.whitehouse.gov/sites/default/files /microsites/ostp/PCASt/pcast_carb_report_sept2014.pdf.

12. Ibid.

13. The White House, Office of the President, "Executive Order—Combating Antibiotic-Resistant Bacteria" (Washington, DC: The White House, September 18, 2014). https://www.whitehouse.gov/the-press-office/2014/09/18/executive-order -combating-antibiotic-resistant-bacteria.

14. The White House, "National Action Plan for Combating Antibiotic-Resistant Bacteria" (Washington, DC: The White House, March 2015). https://www.whitehouse.gov/sites/default/files/docs/national_action_plan_for_combating_antibotic-resistant_bacteria.pdf.

15. Annette Pruss-Ustun, Jamie Bartram, Thomas Clasen, John M. Colford Jr., Oliver Cumming, Valerie Curtis, Sophie Bonjour, Alan D. Dangour, Jennifer De France, Lorna Fewtrell, Matthew C. Freeman, Bruce Gordon, Paul R. Hunter, Richard B. Johnston, Colin Mathers, Daniel Mausezahl, Kate Medlicott, Maria Neira, Meredith Stocks, Jennyfer Wolf, and Sandy Cairncross, "Burden of Disease from Inadequate Water, Sanitation and Hygiene in Low- and Middle-Income Settings: A Retrospective Analysis of Data from 145 Countries," *Tropical Medicine and International Health* 19 (2014): 894–905.

16. World Health Organization and UNICEF, "Progress on Sanitation and Drinking Water, 2013 Update." http://apps.who.int/iris/bitstream/10665/81245/1/9789241505390_eng.pdf.

17. WHO/UNICEF Joint Monitoring Programme (JMP) for Water Supply and Sanitation, "Definitions and Methods." http://www.wssinfo.org/definitions-methods/.

18. World Health Organization and UNICEF, "Progress on Sanitation and Drinking Water, 2013 Update."

19. Pruss-Ustun et al., "Burden of Disease."

20. Ibid.

21. http://globalhandwashing.org.

22. http://globalhandwashing.org/about-us/who-we-are/.

23. http://www.unileverme.com/our-brands/detail/Lifebuoy/333483/.

24. http://ivorysoap.tumblr.com/.

25. http://globalhandwashing.org/.

26. Global Public-Private Partnership for Handwashing, "Exploring New Ideas in Hygiene Integration, Innovations and Insights into Behavioral Drivers," Washington, D.C., October 15, 2014. See video at http://globalhandwashing.org/resources/exploring-new-ideas-in-hygiene-integration-innovations-and-insights-into-behavioral-drivers/.

27. Ibid.

28. http://www.tippytap.org/the-tippy-tap.

29. Global Public-Private Partnership for Handwashing, "Exploring New Ideas in Hygiene Integration" (video).

30. http://blog.soapboxsoaps.com/supporting-nepal-earthquake-victims/.

31. https://www.soapboxsoaps.com/movement.

32. Howard Markel, "Before Ebola: Ellis Island's Terrifying Medical Inspections," *PBS Newshour*, October 15, 2014. http://www.pbs.org/newshour/updates/october-15-1965-remembering-ellis-island/.

33. Centers for Disease Control and Prevention, "Fact Sheet: Screening and Monitoring Travelers to Prevent the Spread of Ebola, Updated, March 16, 2015." http://www.cdc.gov/vhf/ebola/travelers/ebola-screening-factsheet.html.

34. Centers for Disease Control and Prevention, US Department of Health and Human Services, "CARE Check and Report Ebola Kit." http://www.cdc.gov/vhf/ebola /pdf/care-kit.pdf.

35. Global Public-Private Partnership for Handwashing, "Exploring New Ideas in Hygiene Integration" (video).

36. http://www.cute-calendar.com/event/world-hand-hygiene-day/13943.html.

37. http://www.cdc.gov/Features/HandHygiene/.

38. Sheri Fink, "Jubilant Liberia Is Declared Free of Ebola, but Officials Sound Note of Caution," *New York Times*, May 10, 2015, 12.

39. Norimitsu Onishi, "Seeing End of Ebola, Liberia Tries to Repair What Fueled It," *New York Times*, May 9, 2015, 1.

40. Global Public-Private Partnership for Handwashing, "Exploring New Ideas in Hygiene Integration" (video).

INDEX

Achamana ritual, 53
Afshinnekoo, Ebrahim, 14
AIDS, 70, 112
alcohol, x, xvi, 50, 64, 83, 109, 122–23
alcohol-based sanitizers: effectiveness
 of, x, xvi, 27–30, 83–84, 86–87,
 114, 119, 122–23, 134, 181; future
 developments in, 176; and hand
 hygiene compliance, 93, 96–97,
 140–41, 149–52, 159; how to use,
 31–32; when to use, 41, 159; when
 traveling, x, 129–30, 132
alcoholic fermentation, 62–63, 67–68
alcohol rubs. *See* alcohol-based
 sanitizers
Alexander the Great, 56
Alfred P. Sloane Foundation, 15
"Alive and Thrive" program, 171
allergies, 9, 162–63, 177
American Academy of Pediatrics, 31–32
American Public Health Association,
 31–32
American Society for Microbiology
 (ASM), 17–18
amoebic dysentery, 69
anaerobic bacteria, 60
Ancestry Mapper, 13
animalcula, 60
anthrax, 11, 12, 55, 65–66, 69, 156
antibacterial (antiseptic) wipes, 27–29,
 123, 129–30
antibacterial soaps, xvi–xvii, 21, 23–25,
 29, 31–32, 86
antibiotic resistance, x, 12, 24,
 85–86, 165–68, 178, 181. *See also*

drug-resistant microbes; *specific
 names of microbes*
antibiotics, 29, 65, 70, 76, 85–86, 109,
 161, 164, 165–68, 176, 178
antimicrobial gloves, 115
antimicrobial scrub brushes, 82
antiseptics, 3, 25, 28–29, 64, 84–85, 87,
 156
antivaccination movement, 71–72, 161
Antonine Plague, 56
archaea, 11, 69
aseptic (germfree) technique, x–xiii,
 88–90, 138, 152
aseptic packaging, 63
ashes, as cleansing agent, 25–27, 53
"Ask Me If I Washed My Hands"
 campaign, 100
Association of Operating Room
 Nursing (AORN), 82
asthma, 162, 178

Bacillus anthracis. See anthrax
Bacillus subtilis (B. subtilis), 109, 111,
 114
bacteria: antibiotic-resistant, 12, 24,
 85–86, 165–68, 178; benign, 166;
 hand and skin, 2–5; phylotypes
 of, 5; scientific classification of,
 69; in soil, 7, 9–10, 26–27, 45, 106.
 See also microbiomes; *specific
 names of bacteria*
bacterial colonies, 9, 36, 108
bacterial colony forming units (CFUs),
 36–37
bacteriophages, 70